LOOKING YOUNGER--LIVING LONGER

The Art and Science of Youth

Christine Wells
John Redmond

Total Health Publications

TABLE OF CONTENTS

Let's not fool ourselves. Looking and feeling younger is a matter of our physical and mental health. Some people buy youthful looks. Some people work at it. And some people do both. But if we are to do it intelligently we must set out intelligent goals then proceed to accomplish all of them.

We can buy improved looks from our doctors and dentists. Some people go way overboard on this. Some look far worse after their surgeries. Most look better. Some may die. The same is true of other attempts to improve our health. Some people die from over exerting their bodies when they decide they want to look better, feel better or live longer. Of course there are risks to nearly everything we do-- driving a car, eating bacon and eggs, or drinking a Coke or a scotch.

You already know that smoking and high cholesterol are negatives to your health, just as is stress at home or at work. You already know that endurance exercise is good for you. But you may not have all of the best scientific evidence of today at your disposal.

In a recent study of 1000 people between the ages of 50 and 99 in California, in San Diego County, when asked to rate how well they felt on an aging scale of 1 to 10 the mean score was 8.2. You can enjoy aging as long as you accept it. The survey found that people in their 90s rated themselves happier than those in their 50s. There may be some aches and pains and some friends may have gone to that great golf course in the sky, but there are a number of positives. The worries at mid-life have been solved. Nearly 100% of one's time is free to: play golf, read, help others, be more deeply involved in politics, or any number of stress free enjoyable pastimes.

In this book we will look at both the positives and the negatives then you decide what you want to do-- and what you are willing to do. If you decide to lose weight to get back to where you were in your early 20s, the intelligent thing is to make a diet change that you can keep forever. It is worse to go on and off diets than it is to remain overweight. There is no question that keeping our strength up and are weight down is much more difficult at 60 than it was at 16!

Are you really willing to turn down that second glass of Chardonnay? Are you willing to dedicate a few minutes a day to exercise? We all know intellectually what is best. But we are generally "psychological" rather than "logical." The comfort of being inactive and having our bellies full often precludes us doing what is good for us.

In this book we will look at much of the science behind our health. We will include chapters that not everyone needs to read. If you don't use psychoactive drugs, you probably don't need to read about them-- unless you want some knowledge so that you can talk intelligently to your children or your grandchildren about drugs.

We will look a bit at the economics of our health-- where do we get the "most bang from our buck?" What dietary supplements make sense to use, what exercise equipment might be wise to buy, etc.

We hope that we will answer the "whys" and the "hows" of looking good and living well and long. It makes sense to start with the things we are likely to die from—then we will have a good starting point for discussing just how important positive health habits are!

CHAPTER 1
DO YOU HONESTLY WANT TO FEEL BETTER AND LIVE LONGER?

Anyone in his or her right mind wants to feel better and most of us would like to live longer—then why do so many of us continue our bad habits and make our lives shorter and less enjoyable? As has been said, "He who has no time for his health today will have no health for his tomorrow."

Scientists know that developing the right fitness and exercise habits can reduce our pot bellies, eliminate depression, make us proud of our bodies, give us more energy, and reduce our chances of developing the diseases of aging-- such as diabetes, heart problems and high blood pressure, and even cancers. (1) We are all aware that a healthier regimen will enhance our lives. Then why don't we take the steps to do some or all of the things which science recognizes are healthy?

We get in ruts—and you know a rut is a long grave! If mother fed us fruits for dessert we probably continue to eat fruits for dessert. If she fed us pastries and chocolate, we probably continue in that habit. If we exercised when we were young, and enjoyed it, we are more likely to exercise today. But the ease of our 20th century lives makes it so easy to settle into the couch, turn on the tube, and take the easy path to killing time—and killing ourselves. If the only exercise you get is changing channels with the remote control, your thumb may be getting adequate exercise, but your heart is wasting away.

WHAT SHOULD BE OUR CONCERNS AS WE AGE?

Our quality of life must be considered both in health and in illness. That quality can be seen as both our objective functioning, how healthy or ill we really are, and by our subjective feelings about how and who we are. We may feel joy or pain, apprehension or certainty, depression or elation. (2) These feelings go a long way towards our determining that we are healthy. We must be positive about our chances for joy and longevity. More and more people are living to be 100, and the number of centenarians is expected to quadruple within 20 years. Life seems to get better each year and more of us are interested in holding on to this good life. I am reminded of Groucho Marx's lament when he said "If I knew I was going to love so long I'd have taken better care of myself."

If I want to live longer and better I should be aware of what is happening as I age. We're not 20 anymore. At 20 our energy was generally high even without taking proper care of our bodies. As we age we lose muscle tissue. We lose brain cells. Our bodies, at the level of our cells and tissues, do not function as efficiently as they once did. In fact it seems that at about age 50 our degeneration begins to speed up. (3) So as we age it becomes imperative that we exercise and eat effectively in order to both slow our aging and to reverse it.

If we are to be intelligent about changing our lives in a positive direction we should be aware of what is happening to us as we age. When we understand the aging process we can avail ourselves of the programs and products which science tells us will slow or reverse the processes of aging. For this reason, in the next chapter we will look at some of the theories of how we age. In the following chapter we will survey some of the diseases of aging. After we have grasped the realities of what is, or may be, happening to us we can more effectively plan on a fitness program.

We would hope that as you see the potentials for living a longer and more fruitful life you will be more motivated to change your diet and exercise habits—if they need changing. We hope that we can also give you some ideas which may help to improve your mental health and the happiness which results from such a positive change.

You must decide that you want to make a permanent change. So many people start with good intentions. They give up smoking for a few weeks then go back to the weed. They start on a healthy diet then return to their deeply ingrained habits. They start to jog, get some muscle soreness, then retire to the sofa—watching other people exercise.

Don't even start unless you want the change to be permanent. And if you choose to die earlier than necessary just consider that you are doing your bit to control the overpopulation in the world!

Next, you will want to make your life changes as enjoyable as possible. You can watch the television while you ride your exercise bike, jump rope, or walk on a home treadmill. If you don't want to change your diet to include all of the vitamins and minerals you need, you can pop some pills which will give you these nutrients.

If you want to go to a gym, make it a social time—go with your friends every day or two. If you would rather garden or walk—no problem. Just make it enjoyable. Obviously a habit that makes you happy will be a great deal easier to learn than one that is drudgery or otherwise unpleasant.

Dr. William Castelli, the director of the Framingham Heart Study--the longest ongoing study in the world, became the first man in his family to live past age 50. He did it by heeding his own advice of not smoking, restricting fat in his diet, and exercising. At 60 he was fit as a fiddle. And he's going strong in his 70s. My own longevity parallels his. My father died at 48 with an aorta (the main artery from the heart) as hard as a clay pipe and his heart twice the normal size because of the work it had to do to push his blood through that artery. He had done everything wrong: 50 pounds overweight, a 2 pack a day smoker, a heavy fat eating-non-exerciser who lost all the money he had in the Depression. I have just done everything the opposite of my father's habits. So far I have outlived him by more than 30 years. Of course now we have so much more information than was available in my father's day. It's up to you. You can't change your heredity—but you are in control of your environment. You can add years to your life and life to your years—if you want to.

WHAT AND WHY DO YOU WANT TO CHANGE?

We will give you a number of reasons to make positive changes in your life. We will discuss diseases which can be avoided, or at least reduced, with proper health habits. We will give you a greater insight into why you should be more attentive to your diet, your exercise program and your tobacco addiction. You choose which you want to change and how much.

Do you want to exercise just enough to live a bit longer or do you want to exercise to the point where your activity makes positive mental changes in your life? Do you want to lose weight for looking and feeling better or to increase your longevity? Do you want to stop smoking for your own sake or for the sake of your family? We will lay out the facts—you decide if and what you want to do. It's your life!

We will start with the negatives—the diseases and negative health practices. Next we will look improving your fitness by eating a more efficient diet, then we will look at various kinds of exercise programs. We'll try to make it as pleasant a change in your behavior as possible. The rest is up to you!

MENTAL HEALTH

Our mental health is also often negatively affected as we age. We can be more negatively affected by the stresses of business, by changes in our family status, and by the obvious physical affectations of the process of our getting older.

A book on fitness would not be complete without looking at our mental health and the opportunities to make it better—particularly through exercise.

A FINAL THOUGHT

My favorite social scientist and philosopher, Ashley Montagu told us—"that the goal of life is to die young, as late as possible."

END NOTES

1.Shephard, R.J. et al. ''Personal health benefits of Masters athletics competition.'' British Journal of Sports Medicine, vol. 29: pp 35-40.

2.Muldoon, MF. "What are quality of life measurements measuring?" Brit. Med. Jour. Feb. 1998, 316, pp. 542-545.

3. Position statement of World Health Organization presented at the World Congress of Sports Medicine, Orlando, FL. June 3, 1998.

CHAPTER 2
THEORIES OF HOW WE AGE

•To slow aging;
•Consume high anti-oxidant foods and supplements
•Reduce smoke inhalation
•Keep your weight controlled
•Choose your parents wisely
Here's why

We know it's happening but we don't know exactly why or how. If we knew better we would be more able to slow our aging process and live longer and better. Actually we do know some things and these things that we know have helped many people to live longer and more effective lives. Better nutrition, especially eating less fat, and more exercise have allowed many of us to successfully live longer than our parents and grandparents.

If we understand some of the theories of aging that are being researched we can change our health behavior to take advantage of what is known today. But we must remember that aging research doesn't have all of the answers. Our extremely complicated bodies with our own genetic pre-dispositions and our varying environments give us trillions of variables for the researchers to investigate. We may never know all of the answers but we have some ideas.

If we ever completely understand how and why aging occurs the reasons will undoubtedly be a combination of the following theories plus some theories not yet postulated. The theories of aging generally can be classified as ''built in'' or ''genetic'' theories of the cells breaking down or they can be seen as ''damage'' theories in which the genetic material (DNA and RNA) are damaged so that they cannot function properly or reproduce healthy cells. Additionally, when we look at the following theories we can't be certain if aging is a result or a cause of the factors that we observe.

While some wild optimists suggest, based on animal studies, that we might be able to live to be 200, we are a long way from such potential. But scientists around the world, such as those at the Department of Geriatric Medicine at the University of Manchester, are working to unlock the keys to living longer and better. And they are finding that we can each play a part in extending our own lives.

GENETIC THEORIES

Cells of a species tend to multiply and reproduce themselves for a predetermined number of doublings. Once they have completed their predetermined number of doublings the cell stops reproducing so the organism dies. It is assumed that we human beings should be able to live between 110 and 120 years based on the number of doublings expected by human cells.

Studies with some non-human cells indicate that perhaps vitamin E can prolong the number of doublings. Other experiments have indicated that by lowering the body temperature the cells will double slower. If there were temperature lowering drugs, life might be lengthened.

The genetic switching theory holds that the genes have a built-in switch that begins aging at a certain period of one's life. It is therefore similar to the ''cell doubling'' theory

The error catastrophe theory. Deoxyribonucleic acid (DNA) and ribonucleic acid (RNA) are the basic genetic materials. DNA is the basic structure of the genes. It can reproduce itself with the help of the RNA. When either is changed the gene cannot reproduce itself or cannot reproduce itself correctly.

This theory holds that the correct genetic information held in the DNA is changed by enzymes or the environment. This "bad" information is then transmitted to other cells by the RNA. Damage could also have occurred to the RNA which would have resulted in its transmitting erroneous information.

Epigenetics

Epigenetics is the name of the branch of science that studies this. Epigenetics (meaning 'above' genetics) is a relatively recent area of study. It looks at how environmental influences can affect the DNA in a gene--by turning it on or off . (It doesn't change the DNA, one's basic genetic structure, only how much it will be activated in the next generation or the next few generations) It then looks at whether such epigenetic changes can be transmitted to offspring as well as how many generations might be affected by that environmentally changed gene. This whole process is called "trans-generational epigenetic inheritance." It has been studied in plants, bacteria, lower animals and mammals—including humans.

There are a number of factors that can affect the DNA in a gene by turning it on or off. One of the more common epigenetic chemical actions, and the one most extensively studied, is methylation. In methylation a methyl radical (CH_3) attaches to the DNA and affects its ability to control an action.

Scientists are a long way from being able to predict what kinds of external stimuli will produce major or minor affects on which genes. For example there are about 50 genes known to be related to breast cancer that can be affected by the methylation of DNA. It is impossible to predict whether an external stimulus, such as a job stress, would affect any or all of these genes and for how long any changes might be active.

When the DNA is affected, a number of positive or negative outcomes have been observed. Both the attentive grooming of mice or an enriched environment for them can cause positive changes in the animal that can then be transferred to the next generation. But many more negative effects have been found. Stress (which increases various stress hormones), toxins, such as tobacco or marijuana smoke or air pollution, and the effects of both legal and illegal drugs are possible culprits. Depending on which genes are affected, and how they are affected, the resulting combination can affect both the mental and physical health of the newborn.

While the action in the gene is chemical, it can be caused by such things as stress, drugs, smoking, over- or under-eating, or even a happy environment. Depending on the type of gene and whether the switch is on or off, the traits can be transferred in the sperm or ovum and can affect the next-generation of life. It had been thought that changes in the DNA would be reset when pregnancy occurred and that any damage done to one's body would not be transferred to offspring. Now it is found that it is not true and that the changes may be passed on for several generations. In fact we don't know when it might end. One study of corn showed that the changes were extinguished by the seventh generation. But a study of mice found an epigenetic problem that lasted through only five generations.

An example of positive changes can be shown in a mouse study. 15-day-old female mice were provided with a very positive environment, things to play with and wheels to exercise on. When they became pregnant and gave birth, their pups showed very positive personality traits even though they had never lived in such an enriched environment. This was true even when the pups were not raised by their biological mothers. An enriched environment during adolescence, including exercise, resulted in the mice pups having better memories. More social contacts and more exercise change the brain structures somewhat—increasing the number of dendrites at the end of the nerves and develop other positive physical and chemical responses that increase the learning ability and the memory of the mice pups. The changes in this study seemed to last only one generation.

It is much easier to evaluate multiple generational transference in plants and mice than in humans because their life spans are so much shorter. However a study in a rather isolated area in northern Sweden has been able to chart some changes going back 200 years. In studying the effects on males and females during years of slim and bountiful harvests some definite changes in the offspring of the paternal grandfathers were revealed. When prepubescent children had less food, their grandchildren lived much longer. When they had a great deal of food, due to a bountiful harvest, the grandchildren were four times as likely to have diabetes. When the mother had inadequate food there was a positive effect on longevity and on the incidence of cardiovascular problems. This was just the opposite of what occurred with fathers, when their food needs were more than adequately met. Also the children of poorly fed fathers had a lower than normal fertility rate.

Another illustration of the effect of diet on grandchildren was in Holland. In 1944 there was a very harsh winter in the land. The children of mothers who were undernourished had smaller than normal babies. This was expected. What was not expected was that their grandchildren were smaller than normal also, even though their mothers were well-nourished. This probably indicates epigenetic effects passed through the ovum.

A study in London compared sons and grandsons of males who started smoking before age 11. The sons, but not their daughters, had a higher than average body mass index (evidence of overweight) by age 9-- when compared with fathers who had started smoking after age 11.

Metabolic disease syndrome includes a number of negative factors for longevity. It may include: the accumulation of fat around the waist, an increase in the harmful blood fats and a decrease in the good blood fats, higher blood pressure, insulin resistance which may lead to diabetes, and the tendency for inflammation of the blood vessels.

Another epigenetic study found similar metabolic disease symptoms. Chewing betel nut, from the betel palm, is a commonly used stimulant in the world. Between 200 million and 600million people are said to use it. Its stimulant effects are much stronger than nicotine, and it is known to cause a number of negative effects on the person who chews it, including cancers of the mouth and esophagus. But studies in Taiwan indicate that the non-chewing children of the betel nut using fathers have a high rate of metabolic disease syndrome--overweight and obesity.

With this new knowledge we might wonder whether the huge rise of conditions such as autism, ADHD (attention deficit hyperactivity disorder), ADD (attention deficit disorder), anorexia nervosa, overweight and obesity, schizophrenia and other conditions might be, at least partially, explained by epigenetic conditions experienced by the parents and passed on to their children and grandchildren.

If we look back at the last 50 years we can see that one major experience of many youths has been in the use of illegal drugs. Uppers, downers, hallucinogenics, cannabis in a wide range of natural and synthetic chemical makeups. But there is more. Is it possible that microwaves from televisions, computers and ovens might have some effect on future parents of this world. Then there are pesticides, hormonal feeding of cattle and chickens, chemicals and plastics that we're all exposed to and many other possible culprits in the epigenetic list of possible disease causing elements. There is also the overeating by some and the under eating by others. We have already seen how this could affect one's descendants.

It is even possible that the type of food we eat may have some epigenetic effects. A study conducted at the University of Kuopio, Finland, assessed the effect of carbohydrate modification on gene expression with the features of the metabolic syndrome. Eating wheat, oats or potato turned up 62 genes related to stress and had negative effects on biological functioning, such as immunity. On the other hand eating rye products down-regulated 71 genes and up-regulated none.

At Washington State University study with rats showed that two agricultural chemicals, a fungicide and a pesticide, administered to pregnant rats decreased sperm count of their pups and that epigenetic trait was passed down to at least four generations.

There are already studies looking for links between drugs, both legal and illegal, and toxins. We know that high doses of morphine given to mice damage their nervous system. This damage was also seen in their descendants. There are already studies looking at possible epigenetic causes of the autism. While the science of epigenetics is quite new, based on what we have seen so far it might be wise for those who plan to be parents sometime in the future minimize their risks for carrying negative transgenerational DNA. With this in mind it might be wise to consider eliminating any unneeded drug intake and to consider the potential values of organic foods.

Another theory hypothesizes that the immune system, that fights diseases, reduces in efficiency as we age. Problems such as cancers or illnesses therefore progress farther and faster as we age. Appropriate exercise can keep the immune system more efficient, as can proper diet.

CELLULAR DAMAGE THEORIES

--*Free radical aging theory.* In chemical reactions, both inside and outside of the body, non-stable atoms or molecules can be produced. Commonly oxygen, without one of its electrons (a free oxygen radical), attacks body cells in search of an electron that will make it stable. The action of the oxygen radical damages cells. When it attacks the collagen and elastin of the skin, wrinkles form. When it attacks the arteries in the heart a lesion is formed which may then attract the cholesterol which narrows the arteries and sets up a heart attack. When it affects the tissues of the joints arthritis can occur. When it attacks other areas of the body cancers can begin. When it attacks brain tissues dementia and Alzheimer's disease can be the result.

Free oxygen radicals are formed as part of the body's normal functioning, particularly when fats are oxidized in the body for energy. Their production is increased during exercise. Illness and stress also increase their production in the body. They are also present in, or are caused by, air pollution, water pollution, tobacco and other smoke, and sunlight.

A proper diet that is low in fats and high in anti-oxidants can reduce the risk of cell destruction. Reducing or controlling one's life stresses can also have a favorable effect on longevity. Obviously smoke from tobacco, marijuana, or any other source is also a negative environmental factor.

Toxic waste accumulation theory. As we grow older the reproduction of our cells and their ability to repair damage is reduced. This is caused by an accumulation of toxic wastes in the cells. These wastes often become free oxygen radicals which damage the cells. The sources of the wastes are both internal and external. The external sources include environmental pollutants such as pesticides, heavy metals, and radiation. The internal sources are caused by oxidized fats such as over heated or rancid margarine, shortening, butter, or liquid oils.

The cross-linkage aging theory. Free radicals are again involved here. In this theory they combine with proteins in such a way that the cells can no longer absorb nutrients, such as oxygen or water, from the blood. The connective tissues of the body, including collagen (the supporting protein of ligaments, skin, and other tissues becomes hardened leading to stiffness in the tendons, wrinkled skin, and cataracts in the lenses of the eyes. Along with the free oxygen radicals, sunlight, nitrous oxide, heavy metals and stress can also cause cross-linking.

CHRONOLOGICAL AGE AND BIOLOGICAL AGE

The number of years you have lived (chronological age) and the relative age of your body (biological age) are not the same. If your heredity has speeded up your aging or if your environment has created more cell damage you will have a biological age which is older than your chronological age. If you have been stressed, have had excessive free oxygen radical damage because you have eaten too many fats, or if you have been exposed to smoke or other air pollution it is likely that your body is older than it should be.

A lack of exercise can also increase your biological age because that exercise would have increased your immunity to diseases and would have kept your muscles and other organs healthier. It would have also reduced the chances of blood vessel damage through a build up of cholesterol in the heart and brain. Similarly, if you have eaten wisely, had minimized your fat intake and had adequate anti-oxidant vitamins your cells would have suffered less damage because of the lesser amount of free oxygen radicals you would have had.

Biological aging is, to a large degree, dependent on your cells ability to repair themselves as quickly as they are damaged. When the damage occurs at a greater rate than your ability to repair the damage your biological age is increasing.

PHYSICAL CHANGES OF AGING

From the time we are 20 until the age of 75 we will lose:

--about 3 inches in height;

--10% of our brain weight (primarily water),

--30% of our ability to pump blood from the heart (cardiac output);

--65% of our taste buds;

--60% of our ability to use oxygen (maximum oxygen uptake); and

--20% of our body's water content.

Additionally we may:

--become more sensitive to heat and cold;

--lose some bone (osteoporosis);

--develop kidney and bladder problems;

--become constipated more often due to the changes in the musculature of the large intestine;

--become more susceptible to medicines because the liver shrinks and the kidneys become less effective in eliminating wastes;

--lose some mental functioning due to the loss of brain neurons and the lessened ability of the neurotransmitters to work effectively.

SLOWING OR REVERSING THE EFFECTS OF AGING

It is estimated, based on studies with twins, that about 20% of our aging and death potential is set in our genes. That means that about 80% of our aging and death factors are set by our environment—by where we live, and how we live. We therefore have some power over our destinies.

When you understand the theories of aging and the environmental contributions you make to your aging through not exercising effectively, poor eating habits, smoking or drinking, and living a stressful life, you may decide to make some changes. If you will bear with us for one more chapter, on disease, we will begin our expose' of which of our habits may be contributing to our aging and how we can change.

But as we look at each risk factor realize that no one is exactly average. While the average one pack a day smoker cuts his life span by seven years, there are those who smoke and live to be over 100. Of course if we are looking at the averages, there must be a number of people shortening their lives by over seven years if one lives to be over 100.

The importance of the risk factors is also something we may look at. While either not exercising or being obese is the number one factor, the third most important factor of risk is either cholesterol levels or smoking. For the person who has hereditarily high cholesterol, such as a 400 (ideal being under 160 and normal nearer 200), that person will probably not live to be 40—even if he didn't smoke or exercise and was not obese. The high cholesterol level for him became the primary risk factor. Your heredity is very important in determining just how negative each risk factor is for you. However we must remember that the most important risk factors (exercising effectively, being trim, having a low cholesterol, and not smoking) can generally be controlled by us if we merely know where we stand in regard to each one.

For a person with very high cholesterol only medication or an operation can help. Obesity may also need medical help—if it is hereditary. But smoking and exercise levels are definitely behaviors we can control without the help of others. If aging is due to us taking poor care of our bodies, and there is growing evidence that it is, there is hope that solutions can be developed to slow the onset of the diseases of aging. This will be a very difficult job.

The value of a genetic understanding of aging is clear, but interventions need not be genetic. For example, regular athletic exercise is associated with a slowing of the accumulation of mutant mitochondria seen in muscle cells with advancing age. Exercise also reduces blood pressure and overweight and changes the more dangerous cholesterols to the protective ones.

In ancient Rome the average lifespan was about 22 years, now it is approaching 80. In 1850 only one of 6 Englishmen lived to be 75, today it is 4 of 6. (1) We must be doing some things right. The picture we now need to define is of how genes, environments, and lifestyles work together to influence longevity and health in old age. This will not come easily, but come it will if we go at it hard enough. Increasing human life spans to 200 years may take a little longer.

At this point it should be said, loudly and clearly, that the primary goal of research on the biological basis of aging must be to increase the quality of later years of life. If quality is not improved, any increase in longevity would not be a victory. Now let us first take a look at the diseases which are most likely to ''get us'' then we can understand better what we need to do to live longer and better. Later we will look at the mental side of our lives and suggest some ways to make our lives more fulfilling as we are living longer.

AND MORE:

In a large study of older with younger people in China it was concluded that there is a physiological basis for living longer. The major factors included:

a better blood flow to the cells,

a stronger, more efficient heart, lung and circulatory system,

a more effective immune system,

better adrenocortical, liver and kidney functions, and,

a higher level of high density lipoprotein cholesterol.

It was suggested that Chinese traditional medicine, along with Western medicine, might be used to improve the micro-blood-flow, nature killer cell activity, high density lipoprotein cholesterol and vital organ function. (2)

There are a number of signs of aging that become evident after age 25 or 30:

At age 40

--You use about 120 calories per day less than you did at 30 so weight control is more difficult.

--You will be about 5/16th of an inch shorter than at age 30 and you will continue to shrink about an inch every 15 years. This is due to bone loss, the compression of the spinal disks and changes in posture.

--A hearing loss will develop particularly at the higher frequencies. Men have more problems with this than women.

--As the lenses of the eyes become harder there will be more difficulty in focusing on close things, such as newspaper print.

By the 50's

--Muscle cells atrophy and strength is lost.

--Immunity system continues to become less effective increasing one's chances for infections and cancers. This is due in part to the reduction in size of the thymus gland.

--The eye becomes less sensitive to recognizing objects in dim light.

By the 60's

--The joints become stiffer due to less lubrication and the effects of 60 years of use.

--Men's sexual daydreams have pretty well stopped by the mid 60's. The reason is unknown.

--Hearing continues to diminish.

--Diabetes increases as the functioning of the pancreas becomes less efficient.

By the 70's

--The harder artery walls make the heart pump harder so blood pressure increases, usually by 20 to 25%.

--Coordination is reduced probably because of a diminished brain function—often in the cerebellum.

--Short term memory is reduced.

--Half of men show signs of coronary artery disease.

--Sweat glands become less efficient.

By the 80's

--Osteoporosis (loss of calcium in the bones) increases the risk of hip fracture and falling.

--Mental function continues to diminish with about 50% of people showing signs of senility or Alzheimers.

END NOTES

1.Pahor, M. & Applegate, W. "Geriatric medicine" Brit. Med. Jour. 315(7115) Oct. 25, 1997, pp. 1051-1071

2. Department of Aging and Antiaging, Shanghai Institute of Gerontology and Geriatrics, Huadong Hospital, People's Republic of China.

CHAPTER 3
BLOOD VESSEL DISEASES

We should be aware that:
The persistent problems in our age of affluence are aging and killing us.
More than half of our disease problems are caused by us—They are not hereditary.
New medical knowledge can reverse aging
and keep us physiologically young.
Heart attacks, stroke and most cancers have the same causative factors.
If we want to be younger—we had better stay alive—by reducing our risk of dying!
You already know most of the negative behaviors you do and most of the positive things you should do—but maybe not all.
So here is some food for thought!

Most of the diseases that kill us are diseases to which we have contributed. We may neglect to have a physical examination that might have detected an abnormality. We eat too much or exercise too little. Perhaps by understanding a bit more about how these diseases develop, we may decide to change our habits so that we can minimize our chances of developing the problem.

Most people die of diseases which are labeled as chronic or degenerative rather than those which are communicable. Seven of the top ten causes of death are of the chronic-degenerative type which attack us as we age.

The ten top killers are:
Diseases of the heart
Cancer
Stroke (cerebral vascular accidents)
Bronchitis, emphysema, asthma
Accidents
Influenza and Pneumonia
Diabetes
AIDS
Suicide
Homicide

The top four and the seventh are in the chronic and degenerative category. Other degenerative diseases are hardened arteries (atherosclerosis), arthritis, headaches, emphysema, multiple sclerosis, Alzheimer's disease, and low back pain.. These diseases can be inherited or developed by the way we live. A recent 21 year study in Scotland indicated that even our social class affects our chances of developing diseases and dying earlier. The men in the manual trades, and presumably lower social class, died at a higher rate than those who worked in the non-manual areas. (1)

CARDIOVASCULAR DISEASES

The major killer in the Western world is the combination of cardiovascular problems, which affects the heart and the blood vessels of the body. Coronary artery disease, a hardening of the blood vessels which supply blood to the heart, is the most frequent killer of the cardiovascular ailments. Stroke (cerebral vascular accident or CVA), a deadening of brain tissue, is also a blood vessel problem.

In a recent study of male mortality in a number of European countries during the decade of 1980 to 1990 it was found that heart disease was related to manual laboring people in England, Wales, Ireland and the Scandinavian countries but not in Switzerland, France or the other Mediterranean countries—where a number of cancers were a primary cause of death. (2)

The causes of heart attack and stroke are similar because in both cases the blood flow to the organ is slowed or stopped. This lack of blood results in the lack of oxygen and nutrients, deadening the heart muscle or brain tissue. The causes of blood blockage can be a thrombus, a hemorrhage, or compression.

The blood flow may be slowed or stopped by a thrombus, a clot which clogs the blood vessel. It may be slowed by an embolism. This moving clot can slow the blood flow so that the necessary oxygen does not reach the tissues ahead of the embolism. Blood flow can be slowed if the artery is constricted. This can happen if a growing tumor pushes down on the blood vessel. Or blood flow can be slowed if the artery ruptures and the blood hemorrhages.

Heart attack is the most common type of heart ailment. It occurs when an artery of the heart is blocked. The coronary artery or the "crowning" artery of the heart is the major artery of the heart It brings blood to the heart muscle. Without that blood, the heart muscle will not have the oxygen that is needed and will cramp. * This cramping is called a heart attack. The cramping of the muscle occurs in the area forward of the blockage. The area damaged during a heart attack can be so small that the individual doesn't even know that a heart attack has occurred, or it can be so massive that the individual dies immediately.

When the heart attack occurs, there is a scarring of the heart muscle, causing the muscle's death. This is called a myocardial infarction, Latin for "the death of the heart muscle." Once it was thought that the scarring was complete as soon as the heart attack was completed, but now we find that there tends to be a continual scarring and it can spread. This is another reason for immediate expert attention, because effective doctors can minimize the damage that may continue after the first part of the heart attack.

Each year, millions of people die from heart disease. Of these, 65 per cent of the people with severe coronary attacks die before reaching the hospital. But in three out of five cases people survive their first heart attack. Men are more likely to experience these than women, but after menopause a woman's chances greatly increase and her risk is 4 times what it was before menopause.

Strokes are the third leading cause of death accounting for nearly 7 per cent of all deaths. But in people over seventy at least two out of every three deaths are from stroke. Men are more commonly afflicted than women.

A stroke occurs when a blood vessel in the brain is blocked or bursts and the oxygen supply to the brain is cut off. Since the brain requires about 20 per cent of all the blood and the oxygen output of the body, even a small blockage of a blood vessel can do a great deal of harm.

Both exercise and an effective diet can reduce the risks of blood vessel diseases. This is true even with such a serious problem as congestive heart failure, in which the weakened heart cannot pump sufficient blood, exercise can improve the sufferer's endurance and heart strength. Studies at the Free University of Berlin have shown a 65% increase in fitness after only 3 weeks of exercise. (3)

HARDENED ARTERIES AND HIGH BLOOD PRESSURE

Hardened arteries (atherosclerosis) and high blood pressure (hypertension) go hand-in-hand as the major contributors to both heart disease and stroke. Arteries become less efficient when their inner linings thicken and are roughened by these deposits of fat, fibrin, cellular debris, and calcium. The resulting reduction in the diameter of the blood vessels slows the blood flow, making it easier for clots to form and further restrict the blood flow of the arteries. Atherosclerosis is responsible for about 95 per cent of all heart attacks.

Fatty deposits on the artery walls (atherosclerosis) may begin as tumors which accumulate fat. These tumors may result from a genetic defect in the cell. The defect may then be stimulated into growth by outside influences such as high blood pressure (hypertension), cigarette smoking, free oxygen radicals, items in the diet, or possibly viruses.

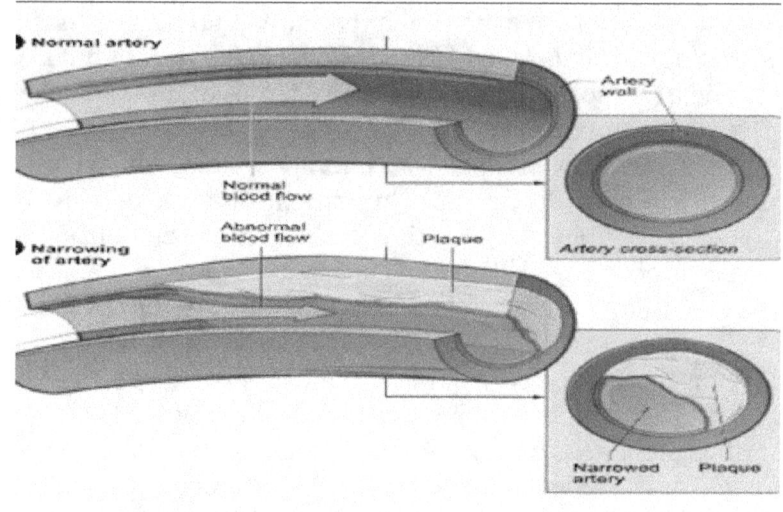

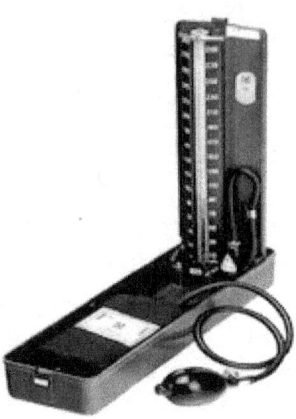

Hypertension (high blood pressure) is the primary indicator of heart attack, stroke, and kidney disease. Many millions of people have it. More than half of them are not aware of their condition because there are usually no symptoms. Blacks are particularly prone to this condition, being afflicted three times more often than whites.

Hypertension is of concern because of the harm it can do to the heart, kidneys, brain, and blood vessels if it remains uncontrolled for long periods of time. The heart is the organ most commonly damaged by high blood pressure. The increased force required during each beat makes the heart muscle thicken and become abnormally enlarged. It also speeds the hardening of the arteries of the heart.

High blood pressure occurs when the blood vessels in the body are constricted, either by nervous impulse or a build-up of plaque in the arteries. The heart is then required to beat more forcefully than normal. This forceful beat increases the pressure of the blood flowing from the heart.

Among the causes for hypertension are: a narrowing of the arteries; a tumor on the adrenal gland; kidney disease; or obstructions in the arteries to the kidneys, and diabetes. These can usually be surgically or medically corrected. Approximately 90 per cent of all high blood pressure cannot be attributed to any one cause. Heredity, obesity, diet (particularly excess salt or inadequate potassium), smoking, and nervousness may each play a part, as can alcohol consumption. Some drugs can also raise blood pressure. Steroids, caffeine, drugs with stimulants (such as some cold remedies, nasal decongestants, and appetite suppressants), cocaine and methamphetamine, and some depressants--because of the rebound effects.

The effects of the disease include: kidney damage, artery wall damage, artery wall aneurysms (bulges) or hemorrhage which is often a cause of strokes, and the development of atherosclerotic plaques in the arteries of the heart and brain.

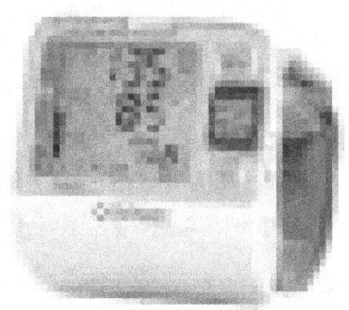

Wrist manometer

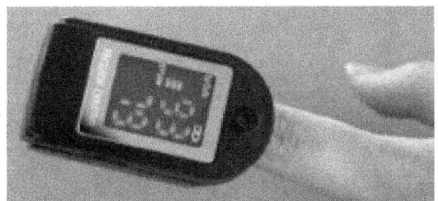

Finger manometer

Your blood pressure is easily checked. You can easily check your blood pressure. Sphygmomanometers (Greek for pulse pressure measurer) and stethoscopes can be bought at any medical supply house. They are quite inexpensive. Some have the stethoscope built into the sphygmomanometer, making it very easy to take one's own blood pressure. Electronic sphygmomanometers are the simplest to use. You can also buy wrist and finger manometers.

The pressure in the arteries fluctuates somewhat. It is higher at the instant that the heart beats. It is lower when the heart is resting between beats.

When taking one's blood pressure the blood flow is first stopped by inflating the air pressure above the measuring device. In a doctor's office it is done in the upper arm and the measuring device is below this area. The air pressure is slowly reduced until the heart is able to force blood past the air cuff. When the force of the heart beat is first able to move blood past the inflated air cuff would have the first measurement of blood pressure − − the systolic pressure. The air pressure is continually reduced until blood can flow past the cuff during the heart's resting phase. This measure is the diastolic phase.

The various pressures are measured by determining how much mercury in a tube is elevated in the sphygmomanometer. A mercury sphygmomanometer is often used in doctors' offices. However gauges are so accurate now that they are commonly used in both doctors' offices and in the home.

Your blood pressure is measured by two numbers. Every beat of your heart pushes a wave of blood through your blood vessels, which raises the pressure in the arteries. This is called systolic blood pressure and is represented by the first number. The blood pressure between heartbeats, when the heart is recovering, is called the diastolic pressure and is the second and lower number.

So called ''normal'' blood pressure is about 110/70 to 120/80. The numbers represent the number of millimeters of mercury that are being lifted in the sphygmomanometer by the pressure of the blood. (This assumes the older type of machine that actually used mercury in a glass tube. Today most machines work with a gauge that gives an equivalent measurement.

110/70 is ideal and is normal for many women, a number of experts would like to have this measure considered to be normal for all. 120/80 is generally considered to be normal and is common for many men. 140/90 is borderline high. Generally lower is better--unless it gets so low that you faint. This may happen when it reaches 90/60 or lower. Some research is questioning the "lower is better" concept because there is some

19

evidence that heart attack risk may elevate when the diastolic level is below 74. (4) Research to determine the validity of this theory and its possible causes is currently being conducted.

Blood pressure may vary greatly during any one day, so a high reading is not conclusive. If it remains high, it may be dangerous--and a doctor should be consulted. Having a sphygmomanometer at home makes it easy to get an accurate picture of your blood pressure. One in six homes already have them.

The danger of high blood pressure can be seen if we understand that a person whose systolic pressure is over 150 has twice the risk of a heart attack and four times the risk of a stroke as a person with a systolic pressure under 120. Insurance companies' studies show that a 35-year-old with a blood pressure of 145/95 lives 12 years less than someone with normal blood pressure.

HOW AND WHERE BLOOD VESSEL PROBLEMS OCCUR

Blood vessel problems occur most commonly in the heart muscle and in the brain. These give us the heart attack and stroke. When there are problems with high blood pressure or blood with an excess of HDL fats, they are more likely to harden the arteries in the heart muscle, because that is where the blood pressure is the highest-- because the blood that nourishes the heart muscle comes directly from the aorta which comes directly from the heart. So the blood pressure here is very high. In the brain the huge number of blood vessels in the brain make it a prime area for blood vessel problems.

A stroke or heart attack happens when the blood flow is slowed or stopped. A clot can stick in the blood vessel and stop the flow. An embolism is a small clot that is moving through the vessel but slowing the blood flow. A hemorrhage occurs when a blood vessel ruptures and allows blood to escape. This reduces the amount of blood in the vessel past the rupture. All of these can cause heart attacks or strokes. An additional problem that is

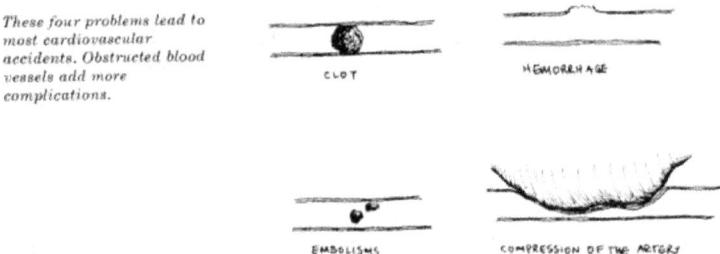

These four problems lead to most cardiovascular accidents. Obstructed blood vessels add more complications.

CLOT   HEMORRHAGE

EMBOLISMS   COMPRESSION OF THE ARTERY

much more likely to happen in the brain than in the heart is compression—where a tumor may grow and compress the blood vessel.

A heart attack is not caused by blood flowing through the heart, but rather the coronary arteries that nourish the heart muscle.

THE CAUSES OF VASCULAR PROBLEMS

It seems that the same factors are related in the development of both atherosclerosis and hypertension. It is likely that either one may cause the other. Thus their possible causes will be discussed together.

Heredity is often responsible for the tendency to high blood pressure and being over-weight. In studies comparing children of both natural and adoptive parents, the parents with abnormal body weight or blood pressure gave birth to children who manifested the same symptoms. Adopted children in the same household tended to have normal readings despite identical diets.

Inherited racial characteristics may also play a part. Among blacks, one in four have hypertension (only one in 500 have the much publicized sickle cell anemia). Among whites, one person in eight is hypertensive. Whether inherited or environmentally induced, our blood pressures seem to be determined, to a large degree, early in our lives.

Environment is a major cause of cardiovascular disease. Being overweight, eating certain types of foods, reactions to stress, cigarette smoking, and inadequate exercise are all possible contributors to cardiovascular diseases.

Exercise that requires that the heart work hard for a reasonably long period of time is a positive factor in keeping the circulatory system functioning efficiently. There are various theories as to why it works, but the results of effective exercise are well established. Exercise aids in reducing the effects of stress, lowers harmful blood fats while raising the protective blood fats, and may increase the number of open blood vessels in the heart. These combined effects not only lessen the possibility of a heart attack, they also increase one's chances of survival should a heart attack occur.

Moderate exercise can improve your heart health significantly. Walking is the activity of choice for many heart patients. The recommended "dosage" is 12 to 15 miles per week, but start at whatever distance is comfortable for you, and gradually increase your mileage over weeks and months. Such exercise can reduce your body weight and blood pressure and can make your heart more efficient by slowing the pulse rate and increasing the amount of blood pumped during each heart beat. (5.)

A recent Dutch study that used 20 sedentary men and 14 sedentary women then trained them by walking and running them 3 or 4 times a week for nine months, culminating with them running a half marathon (13 miles, 21 kilometers) found significant changes in their bodies which resulted from their training. The men lost an average of 5 pounds and the women 2.5 pounds. The men had significant reductions in their total cholesterol, their low density lipoproteins (LDL—the most dangerous of the cholesterols) and their triglycerides. All are greatly associated with heart attack risk. (6) 7) 7. The reduction in risk factors was much greater in the men than in the women but this is partially accounted for by the females hormones which reduce the female risk until menopause.

A British study of nearly 10,000 male civil servants with no history of heart disease followed them for nearly ten years. During that time 474 experienced a heart attack. Of those who had reported that they exercised vigorously (cycling, running or fast walking at over 4 miles per hour) only half had the rate of heart problems occurred. Those who exercised less but still somewhat vigorously, had a 2/3 risk compared to the non-exercisers. The exercise had to be vigorous and aerobic. (7)

Smoking has many negative effects which make the circulatory system less efficient. The smoker raises both blood pressure and blood fats. The carbon monoxide in the blood makes the blood less efficient. This makes the heart work much harder to circulate the required oxygen to the body. Smoking is directly responsible for between 100,000 and 200,000 heart attack deaths each year in the United States and even more in Europe. But five to ten years after quitting brings the risk back to the level of those who have never smoked. (8) In one major study, people who had had heart problems then stopped smoking enjoyed a 62% reduction in deaths over the next 6 years compared with those who continued to smoke. (9)

Excess body fat also increases the work of the heart. Every pound of fat adds about 200 miles of capillaries which must be filled with blood so that the fat can be nourished. Overweight increases the risk of high blood pressure, high blood cholesterol, and diabetes risk.

Stress may be a factor in cardiovascular diseases. The classic study in this area was done by Drs. Meyer Friedman and Ray Rosenman. They brought great insight into the evaluation of stress when they coined the terms Type A and Type B personalities. (10) They cited several characteristics that show up in high-risk heart patients. They found that these high risk people have a chronic and severe sense of time urgency--they want to get things done. There's a constant involvement in multiple projects subject to deadlines. They have a desire for recognition and advancement and an excessive competitive drive. They neglect all aspects of life except work. They have a tendency to take on excessive responsibilities feeling that, "Only I can handle it. " Their speech patterns showed explosiveness and a tendency to hasten the pace of their normal conversation.

The Type A people are excessively ambitious types who show overwhelming aggression, impatience, and are slaves to the clock. They are the competitive types who may even compete with themselves--such as pushing themselves to improve their time while running, jogging, or swimming. They are usually the early-to-bed and early-to-rise types. They drive themselves excessively, skip vacations, walk fast, talk fast, and are compulsive. They're concerned with making money, and they compete in just about everything they do.

The Type B personalities may be just as serious about where they are going but they are easy going, seldom impatient, and they take time out for leisure. They don't feel driven by the clock to get things done. They are not preoccupied with social achievement and are less competitive. This personality type may be easily sidetracked because they are not as intense in their drives to accomplish. Studies have shown that the Type A personality is two to three times as likely to have a heart attack as did the Type B personality.

More recently theorists have looked at the Type A people and concluded that it may not be their hard driving natures as much as their hostility which increases their heart attack risk. The type A's without hostility seemed to live as long as Type B's. But the hostile people seemed to have more heart attacks.

The physiological effects of the negative stress situations are reflected in higher blood pressures and more adrenaline secreted. Both of these are known risk factors for heart problems. Negative stress has also been shown to increase the stickiness of the blood platelets and make them more likely to clot. (11) In the Framingham study, anxiety levels for middle aged men, but not women, was predictive of hypertension. (12) In another study high stress men "out-died" their low stress counterparts by a 3 to 1 ratio over a five year period.

On the other hand, studies at the Institute of Gerontology in Kiev, U. S. S. R., indicate that the easy life may shorten life spans. The studies done there with animals at the molecular level, the cell level, and the systemic level have shown that animals subjected to certain stresses lived longer than those that lived in ideal conditions. Russian researchers believe that the key to long life may be in the hypothalamus. They found that cell nuclei of this gland age at different rates for different people.

Dr. Hans Selye, director of the Institute of Experimental Medicine and Surgery at the University of Montreal, and perhaps the world's authority on stress, said that, "It is not the stress that is the problem, but how one reacts to stress. The trick is not to avoid stress, but to enjoy and master it. "

Stress is often related to not having control of one's situation. Those in the lower social classes are also at the bottom of their job classifications. Those in the bottom 10% of job classifications have four to five times the number of heart attacks than those in the top10% of the job ladder. (13)

Finally, when faced with stressful situations, learn to respond with thought-out solutions and avoid anger and hostility rather than resort to knee-jerk reactions. Recognize that overreacting to things you can't control can be harmful to your heart health.

Hypertension is the price one
pays for being a racehorse
instead of a cow.

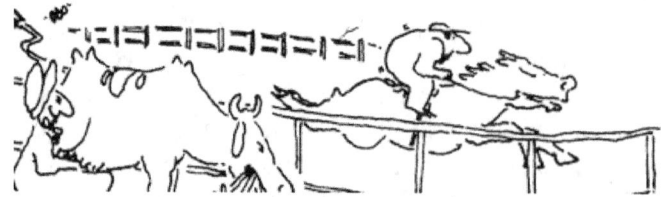

Diet is an area that has been studied at great lengths. In addition to the positive effects of low fat diets and diets low in sodium and high in potassium, the addition of anti-oxidants* is being recognized more often as an important step in reducing both heart disease and many cancers. Vitamins C and E and beta carotene, which is converted into vitamin A, as well as the mineral selenium all have anti-oxidant properties which are thought to reduce the damage in the artery walls which precede the development of the atherosclerotic plaques in the arteries.

People who live in parts of the world which are rich in selenium, a trace mineral found in soil, plants, and water, are much less likely to die of heart attacks, strokes, aneurysms, and other high blood pressure related causes. This mineral is sometimes included among the anti-oxidants. However it has been found toxic in higher doses. European soil is low in selenium so it should be supplemented.(14) American soil is generally relatively high in the mineral.

Moderate alcohol consumption, particularly some red wines, also seems to be preventative for heart disease. It raises the HDL lipids which carry cholesterol away from the tissues and back to the liver. Of course there are some negatives associated with alcohol, the calorie intake is raised which may add body weight and in increased amounts there can be toxic effects to other organs. (15)

Fats in the blood are considered to be prime contributors to hardened arteries. The most studied blood fats are the lipoproteins, cholesterols, and the triglycerides.

The major types of lipoproteins are:

--heavy density lipoproteins (HDL) which transport cholesterol from the body's tissues to the liver where it can be eliminated;

--low density lipoproteins (LDL) which take cholesterol from the liver to the tissues, they contain few triglycerides. 60 to 80% of the body's cholesterol is carried by the LDL; and

--very low density lipoproteins (VLDL) which contain primarily triglycerides with a little cholesterol. They carry triglycerides to the tissues and fat of the body--where they can be used for energy.

Cholesterol is a waxy substance used in many of the body's chemical processes. It is required in everyone in certain amounts. When there is too much cholesterol being carried by the LDLs some can be deposited in the artery walls. This is the buildup which we call atherosclerosis (artery "fat scarring" or hardened arteries).

Cholesterols are derived primarily from saturated fats that are eaten in the diet and from cholesterol which is ingested. About 70 to 80 per cent of cholesterol is made in the body, primarily by the liver, from saturated fats that are eaten; the remaining 20 to 30 per cent of the blood's cholesterol is eaten in the form of cholesterol in animal products.

The amount of cholesterol in your blood is measured as millimoles per liter (mmol/l) in Europe and as milligrams per deciliter (mg/dl) in the United States. To change the Continental measure to the American measure multiply by 38.46. To change the American to the Continental, divide the American number by 38.46.

It is highly recommended that all people have a total blood evaluation when they are young. This can give a "base line" level against which future examinations can be measured. It can also reveal any dangerously high levels of one of the blood fats. The recommended total blood cholesterol level is below 5.19 mmol/l (200 mg/dl) with 3.9 mmol/l (150 mg/dl) being considered to be ideal. Lower is better. In the Framingham study in Massachusetts, which is the classic study in the field of heart disease, there have been 5, 209 adults involved in the program since 1948. In correlating all the factors that relate to heart disease, it was found that the cholesterol levels of the blood are a primary determinant in predicting heart attack risk.

People with blood cholesterol levels over 6.63 mmol/l (255 mg/dl) of blood have five times the heart attack risk as those with the level of 5.72 Europe (220 USA). Men, whose cholesterol level was 5.98 Europe (230 USA), suffered three times as many heart attacks as men with cholesterol levels under 5.46 Europe (210 USA). It is generally considered that for every 0.026 mmol/l (1 point mg/cu. cm3 in U.S.) you drop in your cholesterol level that you reduce your chances of dying by 2%.

High-saturated fat foods, from which cholesterol is made, are found primarily in animal fats such as beef, lamb, pork, ham, whole milk, egg yolks, cream, butter, and whole milk cheeses (the hard cheeses). But they are also found in vegetable fats which are solid or which have been hydrogenated* (trans fatty acids) such as shortenings, coconut oil, cocoa butter, and palm oil (which is used in commercially prepared cookies and pie fillings). They are also found in non-dairy milk and cream substitutes and in chocolate.

While people commonly talk about "good" and "bad" cholesterol it is really the carrier of the cholesterol which is good or bad depending on whether they are taking the cholesterol to the liver or away from the liver and into the tissues--including the arteries.

The HDLs (the good lipoproteins) are associated with lower cardiovascular risk because they are able to get rid of the cholesterols which, if allowed to stay in the blood, can develop plaques in the arteries of the heart, neck and brain. These then increase the risk of heart attack and stroke. Women tend to have more HDL than men. This is caused by the estrogen which they produce. Estrogen replacement after menopause can continue this protection, otherwise women's heart attack rates will rise as they grow older.

While polyunsaturated oils had previously been advocated to reduce blood cholesterol we now know that while decreasing total cholesterol in the blood they lower the HDL. For this reason the monounsaturated fats, such as found in olive oil and canola (rapeseed) oil, are more often recommended as a source for fat.(17) Stopping smoking, maintaining a proper weight, and exercising effectively are all ways in which HDLs may be raised.

The HDL levels should be higher than 0.91 Europe (35 mg/dl USA) for men and over 1.69 Europe (65 mg/dl USA) for women. Higher is better. A level below 0.91 (35) is a very negative risk factor. Another important measure is the ratio of total cholesterol to HDL. It is derived by dividing the HDL level into the total cholesterol level. It should be less than 3 for women and less than 4 for men..

The LDLs (the bad lipoproteins) carry cholesterol to the tissues. Some of this may be implanted in the arteries, hardening and narrowing them. This process seems to need oxygenation in order to occur. It is the free oxygen radicals that change the fat in the LDL. Once it is changed it can be deposited into the artery walls. Both HDL and the anti-oxidant vitamins (A, C, and E) reduce the rate of this oxygenation. (Margolis, Simeon, ibid. p. 5) Vitamin E supplementation of 100 I.U. per day reduced women's risk of heart attack by 33% and men's by 25%. [Ibid]) Dr. Ken Cooper, of Aerobics fame, suggests 400 I.U. per day of vitamin E. The previously mentioned polyunsaturated fats increase the likelihood of oxygenation. The top normal level for LDL is 140 mg/dl, and it is desirable to have it under 130. Lower is better. (See Chapter 9) for more on free oxygen radicals and anti-oxidants.

A Swedish study, sponsored by Volvo, showed that generally women have less LDL than men, but as they move up the occupational scale their levels approach that of men. However while the more competitive type A men had a much higher level than type B men, the type A and B women had similar levels in each job category. The HDL levels for women remained higher than men at every level. (18)

Tri-glycerides are the most common type of blood fat. While they are found in some foods, such as luncheon meats and shellfish, they are generally constructed in the liver from carbohydrates, such as sugars, in the diet. Although we hear much more about cholesterol in the blood, some experts think that the tri-glycerides may be even more harmful than the cholesterols. (19)

Blood tests for tri-glycerides and blood cholesterol should be part of everyone's physical exam from the age of three. The normal level for tri-glycerides it is 1.3 to 3.9 Europe (50-150 USA), but the lower the better. Endurance (aerobic) exercise has been

_____

found to reduce triglycerides (because they are used for energy during the exercise). It also increases the amount of HDL.

Heredity can also play a part in the body's ability to produce too much cholesterol or triglycerides. When heredity is the problem either drug therapy or surgery may be required to eliminate the problem. Even when diet and the lack of exercise are the primary problems, drug therapy can often be used to reduce the blood levels of these fats.

The combination of risk factors increases one's chance of developing a cardiovascular disease, especially coronary artery disease. To the degree that coronary artery disease is increased, the risk of heart attack is increased.

Two members of the Harvard University School of Public Health have reported a study of the health records of 50, 000 former students at Harvard and at the University of Pennsylvania in respect to fatal heart attacks and heart attack risks. The study revealed that 1,146 of the former students died between the ages of thirty and sixty-nine years from fatal heart attacks. When these students were compared with classmates who had not suffered heart attacks, the scientists found six clues or relationships that increase the risk of death from heart attack. These relationships were as follows:

1. Cigarette smoking. Smoking in college was found to be associated with 50 per cent increased risk of a coronary death

2. Non-participation in sports. The college student who engaged in no sports while in college was found to have a 50 per cent increase in his risk of a fatal heart attack.

3. An elevated blood pressure. A systolic blood pressure in excess of 130 mm. Hg. while in college. was found to be associated with a 40 per cent increase in the risk of death from heart attack.

4. Heavier than average body weight. Excessive body weight for height was found to increase the risk of an eventual fatal heart attack by 30 per cent.

5. A height of less than 5 feet 6 inches. Short stature was found by investigators to be associated with an increase of 30 per cent in the risk of death from heart disease.

6. Early death of a parent. The early death of a parent (based on deaths from all causes) was associated with a 30 per cent greater chance of dying from a heart attack.

From this we might infer that the person who smokes cigarettes, is inactive physically, has a slightly elevated blood pressure, is short and overweight, and who has the heredity for a shorter life, as indicated by the early death of a parent, is the person of today who is most apt to have a fatal heart attack in the future.

Other risk factors which have been shown to be related to heart attack and to death from the attack are: depression, anger, and living alone. These factors also multiplied the effects of other risk factors. For example, for smokers who were also depressed, the amount of artery hardening was nearly three and a half times greater than non-depressed smokers. And LDL was twice as high for depressives as for non-depressed people. (20)

You can aid in preventing or slowing of the progress of cardiovascular disease. To slow the hardening of the arteries and to minimize the chances of developing heart disease and strokes, it is wise to keep your blood pressure low and your blood fats in the proper proportions.

In order to begin to do this, it is suggested that you have a physical examination. This will assist in spotting high blood pressure and high cholesterol or high tri-glyceride levels in the blood. It will also find heart irregularities through the use of the stethoscope and the electrocardiogram. For every 1% you reduce your blood pressure or your cholesterol you reduce your heart attack risk by 2 to 3%.

Your eating habits can assist in controlling general body weight, and the lower your body weight, the less your chances are of developing heart disease. You can lower your fat intake. Our average diet is about 35 to 45 per cent in fat. It is suggested that the fat intake be between 10 and 20 per cent of the total calories. Cholesterol intake should be below 300 milligrams per day.

Salt should also be cut down in the diet. There seems to be a direct relationship to the amount of salt in the diet and the amount of high blood pressure. In the northern islands of

Japan, the diet is twice as high in salt as in southern Japan. The frequency of high blood pressure is also twice as high. In Western societies we consume about ten times as much sodium than is necessary, it would be a good idea to take the salt shaker off the table and to avoid highly salted, processed foods.

Vitamin supplementation, while once frowned upon, is now often being recommended. Higher levels of the anti-oxidants, vitamins C, E, and beta carotene and a little selenium are common recommendations. (21)

Taking a half an aspirin daily is also recommended by those who suffer no ill effects from the aspirin. The aspirin reduces the blood's ability to clot so it reduces the risk of a thrombus or embolism forming. A recent study found that after suffering a heart attack or stroke aspirin reduced the chances of a recurrence by 20% and 19% respectively.(22) Omega 3 oil from some fish is also recommended because it reduces the blood's ability to clot and seems to reduce the LDLs.

For normal people one or two glasses of alcohol per day may be beneficial in reducing heart attack risk. But it must be weighed against the possible detrimental effects of increased calories and the possible increase of hypertension. For people who have had heart problems, the drinking of alcohol may be hazardous. Patients with heart disease may be extraordinarily susceptible to myocardial depression (a weakening of the heart muscle action) which is a result of alcohol. Patients with severe cardiac damage and chronic congestive heart failure should probably not drink at all.

Exercise increases the cardiovascular efficiency by increasing the amount of oxygen carrying red cells in each unit of blood. It often lowers blood cholesterol and may widen the blood vessels of the heart. It also seems to decrease the effects of stress.

Stopping smoking is extremely important in the prevention of heart disease. When you stop smoking, your blood pressure will generally lower, the amount of oxygen in each unit of blood will be increased, the artery hardening process will slow, and the amount of cholesterol in the blood will be reduced.

Taking quiet times during the day, which can reduce one's stress, may also be beneficial. Dr. Herbert Benson, Associate Professor of Medicine at Harvard University, studied transcendental meditation. He found that prayer or meditation may promote peace of mind which can reduce stress.

CHECKING YOURSELF

SELF TESTS

Your systolic pressure (pressure at the time your heart is contracting) is the higher number. Your diastolic pressure (the continuous pressure at the time your heart is recovering from its contraction) is the lower number.

Up to 130/ up to 85 is in the normal range—but lower is better.
130-139/85-89 is high normal blood pressure
140-159/90-99 is considered mild hypertension (stage 1)
160-179/100-109 is moderate hypertension (stage 2)
180-209/110-119 is severe hypertension (stage 3)
210 and higher/120 and higher is very severe hypertension (stage 4)
(If your systolic pressure and your diastolic pressures are in different categories, consider yourself in the higher (worse) category.

(Source: Report of the Joint National Committee on Detection, Evaluation, and Treatment of High Blood Pressure, Bethesda, MD, National Heart, Lung, and Blood Institute, National High Blood Pressure Program, 1993)

WHAT IS YOUR HEART ATTACK RISK?

American Heart Association's Heart Attack Risk Test for those who know their cholesterol and blood pressure levels. (Total your points.)

___ Age Men Younger than 35—0 points, 35 to 39—1 point, 40-48—2 points, 49-53—3 points , 54 or older—4 points

_____ Age Women Less than 42—0 points, 42-44—1 point, 45-54—2 points, 55-73—3 points, 74 or older—4 points

_____ Family History Someone in your family had heart disease or a heart attack before age 60—2 points

_____ Inactive Lifestyle (Rarely exercise) 1 point

_____ Weight More than 20 pounds over ideal weight 1 point

_____ Smoking I am a smoker 1 point

_____ Diabetic Male diabetic 1 point Female diabetic 2 points

_____ Total cholesterol level Less than 240 mg/dL (6.23 mmol/L)   0 pints, 240 to 315 mg/dL (6.23 to 8.18 mmol/L) 1 point, above 315 mg/dL (8.18 mmol/L 2 points

_____ HDL level (good cholesterol) Over 60 mg/dL (1.56 mmol/L) subtract   1 point, 39 to 59 mg/dL (1 to 1.53 mmol/L) 0 points, 0-38 mg/dL (0.78 to 1 mmol/L) 1 point, Under 30 mg/dL (0.78 mmol/L)   2 points

_____ Blood Pressure If you take blood pressure medicine—   1 point.
If you don't take blood pressure medicine and your systolic (the higher number) is:
Less than 140 –0 points, 140 to 170 –1 point, Over 170—2 points

_____ TOTAL POINTS (4 points and over indicates a higher than normal risk for a first heart attack.

THINGS TO KNOW

Measuring blood fat levels.

Americans use a cholesterol measurement different from most other countries. The doctors in the United States use milligrams per deciliter (mg/dl). Most other countries use millimoles per liter. (mmol/L) A millimole is a thousenth of a mole.

To convert United States values (mg/dl) to other values (mmol/L) divide the U.S. value by 38.5.

To convert the other values to United States values multiply the other value by 38.5.

So: A desirable level would be under 200 (mg/dl) or 5.2 (mmol/L)

Borderline high would be 200 to 239 (mg/dl) or 5.2 to 6.19 (mmol/L)

High would be over 240 (mg/dl) or 6.2 (mmol

SYMPTOMS OF HEART ATTACK

--An uncomfortable feeling of pressure, fullness or squeezing in the chest

--Possible pain in the shoulder, arm, neck, lower jaw

--Possible dizziness, fainting, nausea, shortness of breath

If any of these symptoms last for more than a few minutes call a doctor

TAKING YOUR BLOOD PRESSURE

To take your blood pressure:

1. Wrap the cuff around your upper arm, just above the elbow.

2. Tighten the screw on the rubber bulb so that you can pump up the cuff.

3. Place the stethoscope on the inside of the elbow, just below the biceps* muscle. (This is where the artery passes.)

4. While listening for a heartbeat with the stethoscope, pump up the cuff. When the gauge shows between 70 and 100 mm of mercury, you should hear your pulse.

5. Continue pumping the cuff until you cannot hear the pulse, perhaps to 140 to 160mm. of mercury. Then slowly let the air out of the cuff by twisting the valve on the air pump.

6. When you hear your heart beat through the stethoscope, note the number on the gauge. This is your systolic pressure (the pressure of your blood when the heart beats).

7. Continue to let the air out *of* the *cuff.* When you no longer hear your heart beat, note the number on the gauge. This is your diastolic pressure (the pressure while the heart is relaxing).

Blood pressure is recorded thus: <u>systolic pressure/</u> diastolic pressure

Normal blood pressure is approximately. 110/70 to <u>120/</u> 80

The diastolic pressure is more important. It may be significant if it is continually higher (Manometers can be purchased from your pharmacy.)

End Notes

1.Smith, GD et al. "Lifetime socioeconomic position and mortality: prospective observational study." British Medical Journal, Feb. 1997 314 p. 547)

2. Kunst, A. et al. "Occupational class and cause specific mortality in middle aged men in 11 European countries: comparison of population based studies." Brit. Med. Jour. 316 p. 7145

3. Meyer, K. Et al. ''Effects of exercise training and activity restriction on 6-minute walking test performance in patients with chronic heart failure.'' American Heart Journal, Apr. 1997: vol 33 (4) pp. 447-453.

4.American Journal of Hypertension, Vol 5 (8), August 1992; Journal of American Medical Assn. Vol 268 (21) Dec. 2, 1992.

5. Spina, R. J. Et al. ''Exercise training enhances cardiac function in response to an after load stress in older men.'' American Journal of Physiology Feb 1997. 272 (2 pt 2) 995-1000.

6. Ponjee, G.A. et al. "Regular physical activity and changes in risk factors for coronary heart disease: a nine months prospective study." European Journal of Clinical Chemistry and Clinical Biochemistry. 34(6) June 1996, pp. 477-483.

7. Morris JN, Clayton DG, Everitt MG, Semmence AM, Burgess EH "Exercise in leisure time: coronary attack and death rates." British Heart Journal 63(6), June 1990, p. 325).

8. University of California Wellness Letter, May 1994, p. 5.

9. Sparrow D, Dawber TR: ''The influence of cigarette smoking on prognosis after a first myocardial infarction: a report from the Framingham study.'' J Chronic Disease 1978;31(6-7):425-432.

10. Friedman, M. and Rosenman, R. Type A Behavior and Your Heart, New York: Alfred A. Knop, 1974.

11. Harvard Health Letter, vol. 2 (5) January 1992, p. 1

12. Markovitz, Jerome, et. al. "Physiological predictors of hypertension in the Framingham study," Journal of American Medical Assn. Vol 270 (20) Nov. 24, 1993. p. 2439.

13. University of California Wellness Letter, May 1994, p. 5

14. Rayman, MP "Selenium: a time to act." Brit. Medical J. 314(387) Feb. 1997, Editorial

15. "Is alcohol good for the heart?" Johns Hopkins Medical Letter--Health After 50. Vol 4 (8)Oct. 1992. p 3

16. Margolis, Simon, and Pascal Goldschmidt-Clermont. Coronary Heart Disease. Johns Hopkins White Papers. Baltimore, MD:Johns Hopkins Medical Institutions. 1993. p. 20

17. Ibid

18. Reported in Harvard Women's Health Watch, Oct. 1994, p. 6.

19. Hodis, Howard. Circulation. American Heart Assn. July 1994

20. "Depression, anger, and the heart," Harvard Heart Letter, Feb. 1993, p. 7)

21. Hertog, Michael, et al. "Dietary antioxidant flavinoids and the risk of coronary heart disease." Lancet Vol 342 (8878) Oct. 23, 1993, p. 1007

22. Anand K. Parekh, M.D., M.P.H., James M. Galloway, M.D., Yuling Hong, M.D., Ph.D., and Janet S. Wright, M.D. Aspirin in the Secondary Prevention of Cardiovascular Disease

N Engl J Med. Jan. 17, 2013; 368:204-205.

CHAPTER 4
CANCER

Cancer causes 16 per cent of all deaths. Half of these deaths will occur before the people reach age sixty-five. Cancer is more than one disease. In fact, it is probably a hundred different diseases. A simple definition of cancer is that it amounts to the uncontrolled growth of abnormal cells. For some reason not yet understood, these cells break away from the normal restraining influences of the body's systems. This uncontrolled growth can impinge on vital organs and block blood vessels by growing to such a mass that tumors develop. A recent theory hinges on the idea that it is not so much that the cells multiply, but that they don't die. A gene has been identified which is part of the immune system and which seems to keep some immune cells alive so that they can "remember" past infections. It is hypothesized that if too many cells are instructed not to die, cancer may be a result.

Tumors can be benign (harmless) or malignant (harmful and spreading). A wart or a cyst would be an example of a benign tumor. Malignant, uncontrolled cancers can either be carcinomas, sarcomas, lymphomas, or leukemias.

-- The carcinomas originate in the linings of the tissues, the epithelial cells such as the skin, the mucus membranes, and the intestinal linings.

-- The sarcomas develop in the muscle, bone, cartilage, and fibrous tissues. These are less common.

--Lymphomas begin in a lymph node.

-- Leukemias are problems in the blood producing bone marrows and the resultant increase in certain white blood cells which spread through the body.

Once a cancer begins, the cells can travel from one place to another by penetrating the walls, the veins of lymph channels. They can then travel with the blood or the lymph to areas that were far distant from their point of origin. This is called metastasis. Many cancers have traveled to distant points of the body before the original cancer is diagnosed. When regional involvement develops there is much less chance of curing the cancer, and if the regional involvement is extensive, death is almost inevitable but not always quick.

Heredity generally does not cause cancer although there is a form of eye cancer which is apparently inherited. However, heredity may predispose a person to cancer. For example, very fair skin would predispose a person to skin cancer from the sun's rays. Cancer does tend to run in families. Several genes have been found which are linked to either the development of cancer cells or the inability of the body to recognize the cells so that they can be destroyed.

Environmental causes are responsible for 60 to 90 per cent of all cancers. Such factors as air pollution, smoking, water pollution, chemicals, foods, radiation, dust, asbestos fibers, and charcoal can be carcinogenic.

The environmental aspects of cancer can be illustrated by the increased breast cancer and leukemia rates of the people who lived in Hiroshima and Nagasaki after the atom bombs were dropped. The leukemia rate (blood cancer) of survivors of Hiroshima and Nagasaki was five times as high as for those people in the Japanese population as a whole. The effect of radiation is shown in the leukemia rates for X-ray workers. It is also seen in the skin cancer rates for people exposed to the sun, such as farmers and sailors.

Chemical agents such as alcohol, cigarette smoke, and soot may have caused cancers of the digestive system, the lungs, and the scrotum. Scrotal cancer is a characteristic found among chimney sweeps in England where they were exposed to the soot of the chimneys.

Only 6, 000 of the 2, 000, 000 known chemicals have been tested for cancer-causing potential. Of these, 50 per cent have already been found to be cancer producing. For example, it is known that there is a link between lung cancer and the handling of asbestos or to exposure to fumes in coking plants. The connection between bladder cancer and exposure to benzene in the rubber and dye industries has also been established.

In 1975, three U. S. scientists shared the Nobel Prize for Physiology and Medicine for their research into possible links between viruses and cancer. But one of them, Dr. Howard Temin of the University of Wisconsin, who did studies linking a type of virus to cancer in chickens, said that he believes that the majority of human cancers are not primarily caused by infectious viruses. It is his belief that the majority of human cancers are caused by radiation and chemicals. The most recent research indicates that cancers may reduce the effectiveness of the immune system in fighting the cancers. So research is attempting to find immune boosters that will not be affected by the cancers.

Certain cancers are caused when normal cells are turned into cancer cells. Very often these cancers need certain amino acids (the building blocks of proteins) in order to grow. When these amino acids, especially phenylalanine and tryptophan, are eliminated from the diet, those certain cancers regressed. However, the elimination of those essential amino acids changed the people's sleep patterns. They dreamed less. They also lost weight because these essential amino acids are needed to build most tissues.

Cancers of the mouth, larynx, esophagus, and liver are definitely related to heavy alcohol consumption. A person who drinks more than three ounces of whiskey, half a bottle of wine, or four glasses of beer a day runs 2 1/2 times the risk of developing mouth and throat cancer. Those who drink and smoke have 15 times the risk of developing cancer of the mouth and throat than those who don't drink and smoke.

Skin cancer attacks 1 in 100 people but its rate has nearly tripled in the last 20 years. There are about 7,000 deaths each year and 32,000 new cases diagnosed. But if diagnosed early, it can be controlled. Usually the lighter one's skin, the greater the danger. This is a reason that blondes and redheads are more susceptible to skin cancer than are brunettes and that blacks, Asians, and Hispanics have only about 5 to 10% of the risk of the lighter skinned people from northern Europe. Australians, who are exposed to 300 sunny days a year, have a very high rate of skin cancers--2 out of 3 Australians will develop some form of the disease.

Skin cancer is the most common form of cancer in the United States. More than 3.5 million skin cancers in over two million people are diagnosed annually.[1]

Each year there are more new cases of skin cancer than the combined incidence of cancers of the breast, prostate, lung and colon.[2]

Treatment of non-melanoma skin cancers increased by nearly 77 percent between 1992 and 2006.[1]

Over the past three decades, more people have had skin cancer than all other cancers combined.[3]

One in five Americans will develop skin cancer in the course of a lifetime.[5]

The worst skin damage occurs to those under 18. Severe sunburns early in life also are correlated with serious cancers later in life. So it is particularly important to protect those who are younger. Young people may have to decide whether they want to look healthier when they are young or when they are older. So you might warn your grandchildren.

While most skin cancers are benign and easily removed, the deadly type, called melanoma, must be taken very seriously. If it is localized on the skin the five year survival rate is 90% but that survival rate drops to 55% if the cancer has spread to nearby organs and to 14% if it has spread to more distant organs.

The outer layer of skin, the epidermis, is made up of several types of cells which can be affected by the ultra-violet rays of the sun. Basal cell carcinoma is the most common type of skin cancer affecting 500,000 people each year. It sometimes metastasizes. Another type of skin cancer is squamous cell carcinoma. There are 100,000 cases of this type of cancer each year. It is caused not only by the sun's rays but also by hydrocarbons found in some oils, tars, and asphalts.

There are several types of serious skin cancers (melanomas). Some appear as darker spots on the skin but the more serious are quite dark, such as moles, and are likely to have a rougher texture.

--Caucasians, particularly women, are likely to develop a melanoma which starts from a normal mole but which becomes irregular in both shape and size. This type accounts for 70% of all cases.

--A second type is more common among Asians and Africans. The lesions are brown-black, blue-black, or dark brown and are likely to occur on the hands, feet, or mucous membranes.

--Another type is most common among women over 50 who have spent years in the sun.

--Another type is more common among men. It starts under the skin. The lesions may appear to be blood blisters but their colors can range from nearly white to blue-black.

A monthly self examination, preferably done with a friend, is the best way to spot an early cancer. Starting from the scalp, check for dark spots under the hair, on the face and neck, in the mouth, behind the ears, on the genitals, as well as on other parts of the body. A common place for such cancers to start in women is on the lower legs, so give them special attention.

The combination of a reduced ozone layer and more recreational hours spent in the sun are responsible for most skin cancers. This makes it more important than ever to wear sun protection with a sun protective factor (SPF) of at least 15. Make certain that it can block both the UV-A and the UV-B rays. It is wisest not to go into the sun when it is at its highest points (from 10 AM to 3 PM) and it is recommended that people not go to sun tanning parlors. The ultra-violet A (UV-A) rays of sun lamps and the sun can cause cancers just as the more dangerous ultra-violet B (UV-B) radiation from the sun, which had been the major concern. If your exercise or recreation program brings you outdoors—jogging, rowing, or lying on the beach—you should take the necessary precautions.

Cancer of the prostate gland annually kills 38, 000 of the 200,000 men diagnosed with the disease. It is the most common cancer in men. In men under fifty, their chances of developing such a cancer are five per cent. In men over fifty, it's 15-30 per cent, and by the time they are seventy-years-old, their chances are 50 per cent. Blacks also have a higher than normal risk of prostate cancer.

Smoking, alcohol use, and particularly the saturated fats in red meat and dairy products are associated with increased risk. Such fats nearly tripled the amount of cancer that would be considered normal.

Men over 50 should have an annual prostate check. In this check a physician puts a gloved finger into the rectum and feels the prostate for unusual lumps. A blood test for prostate specific antigen (PSA) should also be done.

Ovarian cancer is another cancer with strong hereditary links. It kills about 18,000 women annually. With no affected relatives the risk is 1 in 70. With one close relative affected the risk is increased to 1 in 20.

Uterine cancers kill about 14, 000 women each year. The uterine cancers include the cancer of the cervix, the uterus, and the endometrial cancer which affects the body of the uterus. The Pap Smear, named after its developer Dr. George Papanicolaou, is a painless sampling of the cells of the cervix of the uterus. If cancer cells are present, the test detects them.

Cancer cells are measurable long before cancer becomes obvious and impossible to treat. The Pap smear has been responsible for a 65 per cent decline in uterine cancer. It is 95 per cent effective in determining cervical cancer but only 60 per cent effective in determining the endometrial cancer. This endometrial cancer is more likely to occur in older women, and its rate has been increasing rapidly in the last few years. There is some evidence to indicate that the group in which it is increasing the most rapidly, white women over fifty, may be those who are taking estrogen to reduce the symptoms of menopause. It is possible that there is a relationship between endometrial cancer and estrogen.

Women who have had irregular bleeding, spotting, or other vaginal discharges are three times as likely to have a uterine cancer as women with no such difficulties. This is particularly true with women over thirty-five.

Many women have a benign type of tumor in the uterus called a fibroid. These growths usually shrink and disappear naturally after menopause and often do not require surgical removal. For women over thirty-five, a hysterectomy may be the best way of removing fibroids. Other tumors or cysts can occur in the ovaries. They are usually not malignant.

There is strong evidence that the herpes virus, similar to that which causes cold sores, causes both cervical cancer in women and prostate cancer in men. There is also evidence that it can be transferred sexually. One study showed that 15 per cent of men had herpes in their genito-urinary tracts. Herpes transfer can be minimized if the male will wear a condom.

There has been found an 11 per cent incidence of cancer of the breasts and uteruses in wives of men who had prostatic cancer. For wives of men without prostatic cancer, the rate is only one per cent. This indicates that wives of men with prostate cancer should have breast and pelvic check ups every 6 months.

Other correlation's with cervical cancers found that the younger women are when they first experienced sexual intercourse, the greater their chances of developing cervical cancer. Among nuns where you would expect no sexual experience, cervical cancer is virtually unknown. However, widowed women have 50 per cent more cervical cancer than married women, causing us to wonder. Divorced women, however, have 72 per cent more cervical cancer than married women. Jewish women only have one-ninth the chance of non-Jewish women of developing cervical cancer. This is possibly because the Jewish males are circumcised, but there may be other reasons.

Breast cancer will account for several hundred thousand new cases of cancer this year and hundreds of thousands of deaths in the Western world. If found and treated early, the five-year survival rate is 84 per cent. If it is found late, the survival rate is 56 per cent.

Genes that are linked to both ovarian and breast cancer have been discovered. BRCA 1 is located on the 17th chromosome and BRCA 2 is located on the 13th chromosome. These genes may be considered to be responsible for as many as 10% of breast cancers. (1) Yet as many as 19% of breast cancers may have a family history. (2) This study took into consideration not only mothers and sisters but more distant female relatives. Another study while finding that a woman's risk was doubled if her mother was diagnosed with breast cancer before age forty, concluded that only 2.5% of cases involved a family history of breast cancer. This study did not look at the more distant relatives. (3) Another genetic risk is race. Black women have a higher risk than whites until age 40, then their risk begins to drop.

Women who have not breast fed their babies have two-thirds more risk of developing breast cancer than those who have breast fed for at least 36 months. This indicates environmental causes. Alcohol consumption is another environmental risk, possibly because it increases estrogen, (4) as is obesity after menopause. Still 70% of women who develop this cancer have no known risk factors.

While the lifetime risk for developing a breast cancer is 1 in 8, the risk varies greatly with age. For those under 39 it is 1 in 217. From 40 to 59 it is 1 in 26. and for women 60 to 79 it is 1 in 15. (5)

Since two forms of estrogen (estradiol and progesterone) seem to be the culprits, any action which increases their production is a negative and any which reduce it is a positive. So early menstruation is a negative factor since the ovaries start producing these hormones early in life. Having a child and breast feeding it reduce the levels of these hormones, as does aerobic exercise, such as walking or running.

Breast cancers will not hurt, but they can often be detected. A simple breast check for cancer can be done while lying down on the back with one hand behind the head. Curl the fingers of the other hand so that they conform to the shape of the breast. Run your fingers around the breast starting at approximately the "10 O-clock" position. Move the hand slowly around the breast in small and large circles and see if you find any nodules. Some nodules are normal glands; others could be pre-cancerous. You are looking for a dominant lump about the size of a small shirt button or larger.

After you have examined the breasts in the reclining position, examine them in the sitting position. Look for an enlargement of the skin pores or an orange-peel effect on the skin. Feel them for bulging or flattening in one breast which does not appear in the other. Look for a dimpling or puckering in the skin, a sore, a reddening, or a crusty skin. See if there is a change in the appearance of the nipple, especially if it is pulled inward. Squeeze the nipple gently to see if a discharge appears. These breast cancer checks should be done throughout your lifetime since chances of breast cancer increase with age.

The initial cancers are no larger than an "o" on this page, they would be impossible to detect by this method. As they grow larger, they are more easily detectable. Gently feel the breast for lumps or thickenings. Be especially aware of the area between the nipple and the arm pit because this is a common place for cancerous lumps to occur. In addition to this test, you can examine the breast while showering or bathing because the skin is smoother at this time. Either of these checks will be more effective if done just after the menstrual period because the breasts will have lost some of their fullness.

Report any changes to your doctor. In addition to these self-checks, your doctor should examine you periodically. The doctor may use other diagnostic techniques such as x-ray (mammography) or a test for the heat given off by the breast may be used. Abnormal cancer cells give off more heat than normal cells. A new test, called biofield examination, is being tested. It measures the electrical output of the cells. When it is perfected it will be more accurate than the mammogram.

Mammograms, low dose x-rays, are recommended for women starting at age 40 to 50, depending on their risk factors. Experts are not in agreement yet as to whether 40 is too early to start the necessary checks. It can detect tumors and cysts which are too small to be detected by the fingers. Mammograms should be scheduled the week after one's menstrual flow because the potential pain of the squeezing of the breasts during the x-ray is reduced when the breasts are smaller and less tender.

There are seven major types of breast cancers and a number of non-cancerous types of breast problems, several of which will show lumps, thickening, or pain. For this reason a woman should stay in close contact with her doctor regarding any breast abnormalities.

Preventative methods for avoiding breast cancer include making certain that you are getting enough vitamin A and exercising effectively. Women who exercised four hours a week from the time they started menstruating reduced their risk by 60%. Those who exercised 1 to 3 hours per week reduced their risk by 30%. (6)

Men can also contract breast cancer. Each year 1,000 are diagnosed with it and 300 die from the cancer.

Lung cancer takes many lives each year. Its frequency is increasing greater than any other cancer. (There are more than 20 different cancer producing ingredients in cigarettes and cigarette smoke.) Every seven minutes someone dies of lung cancer. It cannot be determined by X-rays until it has passed beyond the curable stage. It therefore must be prevented since it cannot be effectively diagnosed and cured early.

If you are a smoker, the chances of contracting lung cancer are: eight times greater than nonsmokers if you smoke a half a pack a day; nine times greater if you smoke one half to one pack a day; ten times greater if you smoke one to two packs; and twenty times greater if you smoke more than two packs a day. One marijuana joint contains the same amount of cancer producing agents as 20 cigarettes.

In the drawing below you can trace the path of the cigarette smoke down the trachea (wind pipe), into the bronchial tubes and into the tiny air sacs (alveoli) where the oxygen is exchanged in the blood for carbon dioxide which is then exhaled. Emphysema, which is a breakdown of the alveoli, makes the air exchange with the blood more difficult because there is far less of the membranes necessary to exchange the gases from the lungs to the blood. In emphysema, many air sacs are broken and become larger less effective.

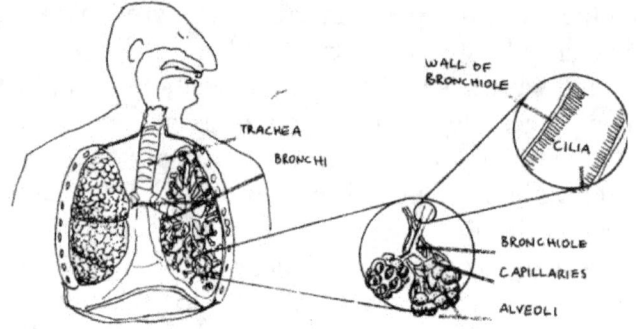

Cancer of the lower intestine accounts for over 150,000 cases each year and about 57, 000 deaths each year. Genetic factors may be responsible for as many as 1 in 7 cases. When detected early this cancer is over 80% curable.

The type of food we eat may be an important factor in determining whether or not we develop cancer of the intestines. Recent studies have indicated that high-fiber diets may move the food through the intestines quicker. This may be a reason that explains that there appears to be a lower incidence of intestinal cancer with people who are on the high fiber diet.

Beer drinking may be a negative factor. Studies have shown a range of 50% to 300% increase in this cancer among beer drinkers as opposed to non-drinkers.

There is now a test to check for inherited factors which contribute to colon cancer. 15% of colon cancers are related to a recently discovered gene. For most people the simple test measuring blood in the stools is used. Of every thousand people tested for such blood, one hundred will have blood in their stools. Of these only 3 will have colon cancer.

DETECTING CANCER

The seven danger signals of cancer are:
--Change in bowel or bladder habits
--A sore that does not heal
--Unusual bleeding or discharge
--Thickening or lump in the breasts or elsewhere
--Indigestion or difficulty in swallowing
--Obvious change in a wart or mole
--Nagging cough or hoarseness

Nearly one-third of those who will die of cancer this year could have been cured if the disease had been diagnosed early. If people are aware of the seven danger signals of cancer and have the appropriate tests done by physicians, their chances of early diagnosis and longer life would be greatly increased.

There are tests that can be medically performed to determine whether or not a person has cancer.

--The previously-mentioned annual medical exams and the self-tests of the breast can be the most important. Mammograms for breasts and Pap smears for cervical cancer are essential.

-- The proctoscopy is effective for finding cancer of the colon and the rectum.

--The barium enema combined with an X-ray may show abnormalities of the large intestine.

-- A test to determine if there is blood in the feces is a method of determining colon cancer.

--The upper digestive tract can be checked by swallowing a barium solution and X-raying it as it passes through the body.

--Leukemia can be determined by taking a white blood-cell count.

--Cancer of the urinary tract can be detected by checking for blood cells in the urine. It has been found that, by using two different types of dyes, the malignant cells, especially those found in bladder cancers, have a strong attraction to one of the stains and become deeply pigmented long before the healthy cells do. This can indicate bladder cancer long before the normal methods would be able to find it.

REDUCING YOUR CHANCES OF CONTRACTING CANCERS

Nearly all of the well known rules for health assist in preventing cancers and other diseases. Avoid tobacco and marijuana, if you drink, do it moderately, exercise, eat effectively making certain that you get enough of the vegetables containing beta carotene and fibers, keep your fat intakes low, keep your weight controlled, and avoid the sun.

AND MORE

Most common signs for skin cancers:

--An open sore which takes at least three weeks to heal.

--A reddish patch anywhere on the body.

--A smooth circular growth with a raised edge and a depressed center.

--A shiny reddish or milky colored bump.

--A pale mark that looks like a scar.

--A wart that bleeds and scabs.

--A mole which is not circular and small. Normal warts are generally less than a quarter of an inch in diameter.

--A mole of irregular shape or with more than one color: including white, reddish, brown, blue, or black.

--Moles that feel rough, that itch, or hurt.

--The skin around a mole that is gray, white, red, or swollen.

ADVANTAGES OF EARLY DETECTION

Among those cancers which have been discovered early and treated, the five year survival rates are these:

If the cancer If the cancer had
was localized: spread to other areas:
Breast 82% survived 47% survived
at least 5 years) at least 5 years
Lung 21% 5%
Mouth 53% 13%
Skin 92% No regional
 Involvement
Uterus 91% 46%

These figures indicate the extreme importance of early diagnosis and treatment.

END NOTES

1."Breast cancer genes" Women's Health Watch [Harvard University] Vol. 2 (4) Dec. 1994. p. 1

2. Slattery, Martha and Richard Kerber. "A comprehensive evaluation of family history and breast cancer risk," Journal of the American Medical Assn. V

3. Colditz, Graham. "Family history from the nurses' health study," Journal of the American Medical Assn. Vol 270 (3) July 21, 1993, p. 338) ol 270 (13) Oct. 6, 1993, p. 1563

4. University of California Wellness Letter, 10:6, March 1994, p. 1)

5. Women's Health Advocate, April 1995, p. 7

6. Tufts University Diet and Nutrition Letter. Vol. 12 (9) Nov. 1994. p. 7

CHAPTER 5
DIABETES

•Diabetes is becoming more common as our population gets fatter.

•Lack of exercise is also a contribution factor.

Here's why.

Diabetes is a chronic disease in which there are high levels of sugar in the blood.

Diabetes affects more than 20 million Americans. Over 40 million Americans have pre-diabetes (which often comes before type 2 diabetes).

Insulin, a hormone produced by the pancreas, is involved. In some people there's not enough insulin, in some there is a resistance to insulin.

Food-- whether, fats, carbohydrates or proteins-- break down into smaller nutrients. One of these, a very simple sugar called glucose, is such an end product. Insulin directs the glucose into muscle cells where it is used as energy, or into fat cells where it is stored for eventual use as energy. When the body does not have sufficient insulin, or is not using insulin properly, the blood-sugar level is too high. This can cause a number of problems such as: hunger, frequent urination, weight loss, fatigue, and excess thirst. More serious complications can include: sores and infections in the leg and problems that may require amputation of a foot or leg, nerve damage.

Type 1 diabetes, formerly called juvenile onset diabetes, is mainly a genetic problem.

Type II diabetes is the most common type and is becoming more common because of high obesity rates in young people. Many affected people do not know that they have it. This is particularly true of heavy aerobic exercisers who are using the glucose for energy—which keeps the blood-sugar level normal even though the insulin levels are low.

Urine analysis and blood tests can determine whether or not diabetes is present.

PREVENTING AND CONTROLLING DIABETES

If insulin is needed the doctor will prescribe it. But we can prevent or reduce its effects by doing the same things we do to prevent blood vessel and cancer problems— exercise, control of weight and eating intelligently.

Staying alive and well starts with food.

We have been eating so long that we think we know all about it.

Enough good foods lengthen our lives.

Too much bad food shortens our life or makes it less enjoyable..

With food labeling required on most foods, we should be able to choose our foods more effectively.

You don't want to eat yourself into the grave.

A little knowledge goes a long way!

Here are the basics--

The next chapters deal with the basic nutrients we must consume. Effective nutrition is critical for diabetics. The next three chapters will deal with: vitamins and minerals, the types of foods we eat and some things that we should consider relative to our eating habits and managing our weight, as well as some recent research on supplementing our diets. While we must obtain our nutrients we also may be interested in taste, our weight, and other elements that we, in the 21st Century, have found to be both delights and problems.

As we age our nutritional needs may change. We need fewer calories to maintain our weight. Our diets may become less nutritious, yet our bodies may need higher levels of some nutrients to ward off diseases. So we must be aware of what is needed and how to get what we need.

CHAPTER 6 NUTRITION

A basic understanding of the science of nutrition is essential to healthy living. An informed person will be aware of the nutrients necessary for minimal function, then put that knowledge into practice by developing a proper diet. Unfortunately, very few people consume even the minimum amounts of all nutrients. They may be shy in protein, fat, carbohydrates, vitamins, minerals, fiber, or water (the essential non-nutrient).

The first three nutrients listed (protein, fat, and carbohydrates) bring with them the energy required to keep us alive in addition to their specific contributions to the body that will be discussed in detail later. All of the food energy that we consume comes in the form of calories. The last four nutrients do not bring with them calories when consumed.

The calorie used in counting food energy is really a kilocalorie, one thousand times larger than the calorie commonly used as a measurement of heat in chemistry classes. In one food calorie (kilocalorie), there is enough energy to heat 1 kilogram of water 1 degree Celsius, or to lift 3,000 pounds of weight one foot high. So those little calories you see listed on the cookie packages you buy pack a lot of energy.

In the more scientific literature, food energy is often listed in terms of joules or kilojoules (kJ). The joule is a measure of work rather than a measure of heat. To convert a kilocalorie into its kilojoule equivalent multiply it by 4.2. In this book we will use the measure of calories since it is still commonly used by most people.

Most people need about 10 calories per pound just to stay alive. If you plan to do something other than just lie in bed all day, you may need about 17 calories per pound of body weight per day in order to keep yourself going. The starvation level for the average person is around 1300 calories per day.

PROTEIN

Protein is made up of 22 amino acids, otherwise known as the "building blocks of life." Amino acids are made up of carbon, hydrogen, oxygen, and nitrogen. While both fats and carbohydrates contain the first three elements, nitrogen is found only in protein. Protein is essential for building nearly every part of the body -- the brain, heart, organs, skin, muscles, and even the blood.

There are 4 calories in one gram of protein, although there are measures indicating that it is 5.6 calories. Adults require .75 grams of protein per kilogram of body weight per day, unless one's body utilizes more protein, as is the case with muscular dystrophy patients. This translates into one-third a gram of protein per pound of body weight. So, an easy estimate for your protein requirements in grams per day would be to divide your body weight by 3. For instance, if you weigh 150 pounds, you need about 50 grams of protein per day. The elderly may require as much protein per day as do children (1.15 gms. per day) due to their decreased energy intake coupled with their possible decreased utilization of dietary protein

Physically active adults have been thought to require more protein than is recommended by the Recommended Daily Allowance (USRDA), which is set at .8 grams per kilogram of body weight per day. In fact, most active people need not eat additional protein if they keep 12-15% of their total calories as protein. Since active individuals need to consume more calories per day than their inactive counterparts due to their increased energy expenditure, active adults who keep their protein intake around 15% of their total calories will eat more protein per day and thereby fulfill their body's protein requirement. (1) Excess protein consumption (above the body's requirement) will be broken down and the calories will either be burned off or stored as fat.

However, when involved in a strenuous strength training regimen, it may be necessary to increase your protein intake percentage depending on the amount of total calories you consume per day. Strength trained athletes have been shown to adapt to diets considered low in protein (.86 grams per kilogram per day) by decreasing their overall body protein synthesis. This is not a good idea since the purpose of strength training is to build muscle, and you don't want to do anything to hamper this process. Therefore, those who participate in heavy resistance training may choose to follow a diet higher in protein (1.4 grams per kilogram per day) to elicit maximum benefits from their workout (2) This increased protein demand also appears true for novice bodybuilders who trained intensively (1.5 hours per day, 6 days per week) for one month

In order to make anything in your body, including muscle, you must first have all of the necessary amino acids. Some of them your body can manufacture, while others you must get from your food. Those amino acids that you must get from your food are called the essential amino acids, while the others that you can make are known as the non-essential amino acids. During childhood, 9 of the 22 amino acids are essential, while in adulthood we acquire the ability to synthesize one additional amino acid, leaving us with 8 essential amino acids.

Amino acids cannot be stored in the body. Therefore, people need to consume their minimum amounts of protein every day. If adequate protein is not consumed, the body immediately begins to break down tissue (usually beginning with muscle tissue) to release the essential amino acids. If even one essential amino acid is lacking, the other essential ones are not able to work to their capacities. For example, if methionine (the most commonly-lacking amino acid) is present at 60 percent of the minimum requirement, the other seven essential amino acids are limited to near 60 percent of their potential. When they are not used, amino acids are de-aminated and excreted as urea in the urine.

Animal products (i.e. fish, poultry, and beef) and animal by-products (i.e. milk, eggs, cheese) are rich in readily usable protein. This means that when you eat animal products or by-products, the protein you consume can be converted into protein in your body because these sources have all of the essential amino acids in them. These foods are called complete protein sources.

Incomplete protein sources are any other food sources that provide protein but not all of the essential amino acids. Some examples of incomplete proteins include beans, peas, and nuts. These food sources must be combined with other food sources that have the missing essential amino acids so that you can make protein in your body. Some examples of complimentary foods are rice and beans, or peanut butter on whole wheat bread.

The essential amino acids and some foods in which they are contained:
Iso-leucine: fish, beef, organ meats, eggs, shellfish, whole wheat, soya, milk.
Leucine: beef, fish, organ meats, eggs, soya, shellfish, whole wheat, milk, liver.
Lysine: fish, beef, organ meats, shellfish, eggs, soya, milk, liver .
Methionine*: fish, beef, shellfish, eggs, milk, liver, whole wheat, cheese.
Phenylalanine: beef, fish eggs, whole wheat, shellfish, organ meats, soya, milk.
Threonine: fish, beef, organ meats, eggs, shellfish, soya, liver .
Tryptophan: soy milk, fish, beef, soy flour, organ meats, shell fish, eggs.
Valine: beef, fish, organ meats, eggs, soya, milk, whole wheat, liver.
*Cystine (sis'ten). A non-essential amino acid that can be ingested or can be made from methionine; thus, the two are often listed together.

The most common protein foods were ranked according to protein quality by the Food and Agricultural Organization of the United Nations in 1957 and revised in 1973. (3). The higher the rating, the better the essential amino acid ratio -- that is, more of the essential amino acids are present. According to the ranking,

Biological value Amino acid score (FAO/WHO)
whole eggs 94% 100%
cow's milk 84% 98
fish 83% 100
beef 74% 100
soybeans 73% 63
brown rice 73% 59

white potatoes 67% 48
whole grain wheat 65% 45
 beans 58% 46
 peanuts 54%. 55

Another reason to be aware of specific food combinations is to enhance the absorption of the protein consumed. The person who is aware of the varying qualities of proteins can combine them to take advantage of the strengths of each. For example, if flour is eaten at breakfast (i.e., as a piece of toast or coffee cake) and washed down with coffee, and then a glass of milk is consumed at lunch, each of the protein sources would be absorbed by the body at a lower potential. But if the bread was consumed with the milk at either meal, the higher protein values of both would be absorbed by the body immediately.

Not all protein sources are equally good. The most common protein foods were ranked according to protein quality by the Food and Agricultural Organization of the United Nations in 1957 and revised in 1973. The higher the rating, the better the essential amino acid ratio -- that is, more of the essential amino acids are present. According to the ranking, whole eggs have the highest quality of protein, its biological value) with a ranking of 94%. Cow's milk is second with a biological rating of 84%; fish rate an 83% rating and beef rates 74%.

The Food and Agricultural Organization has rated each amino acid in food.refined their findings by rating the quantity of each amino acid in a food. Here is an example of the rankings based on the percentages of three of the essential amino acids:

	Lysine	Methionine (and cystine)	Tryptophan
Hen's egg	167	138	107
Cow's milk	169	79	100
Soybeans	167	67	100
White wheat flour	55	105	86
Mixture of 1/3 milk and 2/3 flour	93	95	93
Mixture of 1/3 soy- bean and 2/3 flour	93	93	93

From the above chart, you can see that even the highly rated milk or soybeans are relatively low in methionine and cystine. But if we combined them with wheat flour, we can bring their protein quality into the 93 to 95 range. And the flour, which rated 86% in tryptophan, was raised to 93%.

It should be noted that in eggs 56% of the protein and 20% of the calories are in the egg white, while all of the fat and cholesterol is in the egg yolk. Similarly skim milk actually yields more protein than whole milk at only half of the calories—and with no fat.

Protein supplements are used by some people, particularly weight trainers and athletes. They may be dangerous. Infants under one year of age and older people with liver or kidney ailments often cannot handle the highly concentrated doses of protein in the commercially prepared supplements. These supplements may not be a good value because they usually fall far short of a good balance of the essential amino acids. While six of the essential amino acids are usually present in good quantities in these supplements, methionine and tryptophan are usually found in lesser amounts. Since 910 milligrams of methionine and 245 milligrams of tryptophan are the recommended daily allowances, you might check to determine how much of these are actually contained in a supplement. This is especially important if your diet is lacking in either one or both of these amino acids and you are primarily relying on the supplement to account for most or all of your protein needs. A better and cheaper source of protein for one needing a supplement would be powdered milk. If your diet is deficient in protein, you might consider using egg whites (or egg substitutes), milk, fish or chicken. It may prove less expensive and more nutritious.

FAT

Fat is made of carbon, hydrogen and oxygen. There are 9.4 calories in a gram of fat. In the body, fat is used to develop the myelin sheath that surrounds the nerves. It also aids in the absorption of vitamins A, D, E, and K, which are the fat-soluble vitamins. It serves as a protective layer around our vital organs, and it is an insulator against the cold. It is also an outstanding concentrated energy source. And, of course, its most redeeming quality is that it adds flavor and juiciness to food!

Just as protein is broken down into different kinds of nitrogen compounds called amino acids, there are also different kinds of fats. There are three major kinds of fats (fatty acids): saturated fats, monounsaturated fats, and polyunsaturated fats.

Saturated fats are "saturated" with hydrogen atoms. They are generally solid at room temperature and are most likely found in animal fats, egg yolks, and the cream in whole milk products. They are also found in the commonly used palm kernel oil and coconut oil. These inexpensive oils are commonly found in commercial baked goods such as cookies and crackers. Since these are the fats that are primarily responsible for raising the blood cholesterol level and hardening the arteries, they should be minimized in your diet. Always read the food label..

Monounsaturated fats (oleic fatty acids) have room for two hydrogen ions to double bond to one carbon. They are liquid at room temperature and are found in great amounts in olive, peanut, and rapeseed (canola) oils. Dietary monounsaturated fats have been shown to have the greatest effect on the efflux of cholesterol, thereby reducing the tendency of the arteries to harden.

Polyunsaturated fats (linoleic fatty acids) have at least two carbon double bonds available, which translates into space for at least four hydrogen ions. Polyunsaturated fats are also liquid at room temperature and are found in the highest proportions in vegetable sources and fatty fish. Safflower, corn, and linseed oils are good sources of this type of fat. Polyunsaturated fatty acids of the omega-3 type have been shown to be valuable in the prevention of atherosclerosis. They may even reverse the build-up of arterial plaques.

Omega 3 fatty acids are being shown to be valuable in a number of areas, particularly in the prevention and treatment of blood vessel diseases. They reduce the fibrin, which is a clotting agent, so they reduce clots and embolisms and make the blood flow more freely. This has one disadvantage in the brain where the reduced clotting ability may make a brain hemorrhage worse. They also seem to reduce serum triglycerides and may be helpful for diabetics.

They have also been shown to reduce pain from rheumatoid arthritis and to be positive factors in some cancer treatments and some studies indicate that they reduce the risk of breast cancer. There is also evidence that they may lessen the risk of Alzheimer's disease, depression and schizophrenia..

The omega-3 fatty acids are commonly found in plants such as grass, flax, seaweed and algae. These fats cannot be synthesized in the body so they are considered to be essential fatty acids. Fish are more likely to consume these omega 3s, so they are higher in these fats than are land animals. Fatty fish, having more fat, are the best form of omega 3 oils. These oils are very high in salmon, ocean trout, mackerel, sardines and herring. Of the land animals, grass fed sheep and cows have more omega 3s than grain fed animals. (4)

In addition to omega 3 fatty acids there are also omega 6 and omega 9 fatty acids. Some of the essential fats in your body can be made from other fats that you consume. Those that your body cannot make are called essential fatty acids. Each of these fatty acids, omega-3, 6 and 9 are combinations of other fatty acids. Alpha-linolenic acid (ALA), an omega-3 fatty acid, and linoleic acid (LA), an omega-6 fatty acid, are considered essential fatty acids because they cannot be synthesized by humans. The omega 9 fatty acids can normally be synthesized in the body so are not of major importance to us.

While omega 3 and omega 6 fatty acids are necessary for the formation and maintenance of cell membranes and brain tissue. A problem can occur when there is an excess of omega 6s compared to the omega 3s. Pain producing prostaglandins can result. Many of us, with our modern diets containing so many vegetable oils, may get increased pain in our muscles and joints. Ideal fat ratios are estimated to be between a 1 to 1 and a 4 to 1 ratio of omega 3 to omega 6. But most of us have ratios of 10 to 1 and even 40 to 1 of omega 6s to 3s. For this reason we are advised to eat fish oils or supplement with fish oil pills (5) and use flaxseed oil in salads. But cooking with flaxseed oil is not recommended because it oxidizes (produces free oxygen radicals) at a fairly low temperature. Below are the omega 3 and 6 ratios in some common

Oil	Omega-6 Content	Omega-3 Content
Safflower	75%	0%
Sunflower	65%	0%
Corn	54%	0%
Cottonseed	50%	0%
Sesame	42%	0%
Peanut	32%	0%
Soybean	51%	7%
Canola	20%	9%
Walnut	52%	10%
Flaxseed	14%	57%
Fish*	0%	100%

oils. Since the recommended amounts are considered to be between equal amounts of the two to four times as much omega-3s as omega-6s, you can see by the chart, the ratios in common oils of omega-6 to omega -3 ratios are: canola 2:1 and soybean 7:1, but flax oil is 1 to 3. Other negative ratios for oils are: olive oil 13 to 1, corn oil 46 to 1, while sunflower, cottonseed and peanut oils have only infinitesimal amounts of omega 3s.

Daily Needs

The recommended intake of omega 3 fatty acids is 1.6 grams per day for men and 1.1 for women. They are recommended to be 0.6 to 1.2% of total calories. The American Heart Association recommends eating oily fish or fish oil supplements twice a week. For those with coronary artery disease it recommends one gram of EPA and DHA per day. For those desiring to lower blood triglycerides it recommends 2 to 4 grams per day in supplements.

Here are the amounts of omega-3s in fish. For a 3 ounce (85 gram) serving: herring and sardines have about 1.8 grams of omega 3s. Mackerel and salmon about 1.5g, halibut 1.8, tuna 0.7, canned tuna 0.2, cod and catfish 0. 2, pollack and flounder 0.45. Plant sources of omega 3s are: kiwi fruit 63%, flax 60%, walnuts 6%, and hazel nuts 1%.

Just as the percentage of each amino acid varies in different types of foods, the amounts and percentages of the different types of fats vary from food to food.

We eat too much fat. The minimum requirement for fat in the diet is considered to be somewhere between 10 and 20 percent of the total calories consumed. The absolute maximum should be 30 percent, which is the amount now recommended for the Western diet. While we, as a society, are still above this 30 percent value, we have been declining since the 1970s, so let's try to keep that trend going. Most of us consume between 35 and 50 percent of our total calories in fats. Also, our typical diet is very high in saturated fats, and these are the fats that we want to avoid. If we hadn't been too careful about this in our youth it is time now to change for the better.

Our high fat intake, most of which is saturated, tends to raise blood cholesterol levels in many people. For those who are interested in decreasing the chances of developing hardened arteries by lowering their blood cholesterol level, it is recommended that you follow a diet low in fat (with the saturated fat intake at 10 percent or less of the total diet) and consume less than 300 milligrams of cholesterol daily. Put another way, keep the total calories from fat under a third of your total intake and eat twice as much polyunsaturated and monounsaturated fats as saturated fat.

A recent study, which summarized a large number of studies, indicates that "in typical British diets replacing 60% of saturated fats by other fats and avoiding 60% of dietary cholesterol would reduce blood total cholesterol by about 0.8 mmol/l (that is, by 10-15%), with four fifths of this reduction being in low density lipoprotein cholesterol." That is the "bad" cholesterol. (6)

In the past, companies were allowed to merely identify the oil in a product on their labels as vegetable oil; under the more recent requirements, they are now required to note whether it is corn oil, cottonseed oil, soybean oil, etc., because some of the oils, even though they are not of animal origin, are very high in saturated fat. Palm kernel oil and coconut oil are particularly high in saturated fats. Some countries are still allowed to state on their food packages that the product contains one of several oils such as: "contains one of the following oils: canola, soy, or palm kernel oil." When this is listed you can pretty well bet that the oil is the harmful palm kernel oil. The others are more expensive.

As can be seen from the previous chart, corn oil or safflower oil margarines are far better than butter in terms of the ratio of polyunsaturated to saturated fats. Butter has 17 grams of saturated fat to one gram of polyunsaturated fat while safflower margarine has one gram of saturated fat to 2 1/2 grams of polyunsaturated fat. The margarine is obviously far better in terms of its ratio of fat, but both margarine and butter contribute to the total fat intake. In addition, in order to make margarine stay solid at room temperature, hydrogen gas is bubbled through the oil to chemically saturate the open bonds. This then leaves you with a chemically saturated polyunsaturated fat! The harder the margarine (ie. stick form), the more it has been through the hydrogenation process and the more chemically saturated polyunsaturated fats you have in the margarine. The result of this is that your blood trans-fatty acid levels increase with consumption of this type of fat, and the risks of this are still being explored. So, while we know that saturated fat increases blood cholesterol which, in turn, increases your risk of heart disease, the consumption of margarine may also be a risk factor in heart disease and cancers due to the trans-fatty acids.

When buying foods, especially cookies and crackers, always check the type of fat used. Avoid those with palm kernel oil and coconut oil. Also be aware of the hydrogenated oils used. While a hydrogenated safflower or canola oil may still have an acceptable fat ratio, a hydrogenated peanut or cottonseed oil may not contain the desired levels of unsaturated fats. Partially hydrogenated vegetable oils may contribute to the development of heart disease. The dietary use of hydrogenated corn oil stick margarine increased LDL cholesterol levels when compared to the use of similar amounts of corn oil, also indicating an increased risk of heart disease through the use of hydrogenation (7)

Eggs, which are another staple in the average diet, contain a great deal of cholesterol and saturated fat in the yolk. The American Heart Association suggests that no more than four egg yolks be eaten per week. This includes egg yolks that are hidden in other foods, such as cakes, custards, bread, noodles, and waffles. An egg yolk contains nearly 300 milligrams of cholesterol, which is the recommended daily *maximum* for cholesterol intake. In addition, the saturated fat in the yolk contributes to one's blood cholesterol profile in a negative way. So, while the egg white is a good source of protein in the diet, the egg yolk is something to be avoided.

In order to allow us to have our scrambled eggs without contributing to our risk of heart disease, some companies have developed a low-cholesterol egg substitute. Since most of the cholesterol is found in the yolks of the eggs, they have removed the yolk and substituted corn oil, nonfat dry milk, and other additives. This drops the cholesterol level of one egg from 275 milligrams to less than one milligram of cholesterol. The egg substitute can also be used in cooking where eggs are required. Egg substitutes can be found in the frozen food or the egg sections at the market. If you do your own baking it is recommended that rather than using a whole egg in a recipe, use an egg substitute or replace one egg with two egg whites and throw away the yolks.

Whole milk, another diet staple, contains 3 1/2 percent fat, accounting for nearly half of its total calories. Low fat milk has between one and two percent fat . Whole milk contains 320 calories from fat per quart and low fat milk contains about 184 calories from fat per quart, while nonfat milk has minimal, if any, fat. But each type of milk contains about the same amount of protein (145 calories from protein and 200 calories from carbohydrates). So skim milk or nonfat milk is obviously far superior as a high-protein, low-calorie, no fat food.

Cholesterol in the diet is not as important as saturated fats in the diet in terms of controlling one's blood cholesterol level. For this reason, saturated fats should be reduced. This means that the major sources of saturated fats (red meats, butter, egg yolks, chicken skin, and other animal fats) should be greatly decreased. As an informed consumer you may want to keep track of both your total fat intake and your intake of saturated fat to become better aware of your potential risk for heart disease. For example, one egg contains 5.6 grams of fat and only 0.7 grams of polyunsaturated fat but 275 mg of cholesterol while an equal weight of ground beef contains 8.7 grams of fat and only 0.4 grams of polyunsaturated fats and 45 mg of cholesterol.

It may be possible to reverse the arterial fat build-up through a diet that is very low in fat. Experiments with monkeys have shown that the artery plaque could be developed by a high saturated fat diet. When the monkeys were given a low-fat, low-cholesterol diet for 18 months, 50 percent of the plaque build-up disappeared. After results from these studies were made public, human studies were begun. A very low-fat diet or through medication and diet modification, artery plaque build-up can be reversed (8). However if it has become ''calcified,'' which often occurs with advancing age, it cannot be reduced.

CARBOHYDRATES

Carbohydrates are made from carbon, hydrogen, and oxygen, just as are fats, but carbs are generally a simpler type of molecule. There are four calories in a gram of carbohydrate. If not utilized immediately for energy as sugar (glucose), they are either stored in the body as a sugar called glycogen (the stored form of glucose) or synthesized into fat and stored. Some carbohydrates cannot be broken down by the body's digestive processes. These are called fibers and will be discussed later. Of the digestible carbohydrates, we will separate them into two categories: simple and complex. Simple carbohydrates are the most readily usable energy source in the body and include such things as sugar, honey, and fruit. Complex carbohydrates are the starches. Complex carbs also break down into sugar for energy, but their breakdown is slower than with simple carbs. Also, complex carbohydrates bring with them various vitamins and minerals.

People often eat too many simple carbohydrates. These are the so-called "empty calories." They are empty because they have no vitamins, minerals, or fibers. While a person who uses a great deal of energy can consume these empty calories without potential weight gain, most of us find these empty calories settling on our hips. The average person consumes 125 pounds of sugar per year, which is equivalent to one teaspoon every 40 minutes, night and day. Since each teaspoon of sugar contains 17 calories, this amounts to 231,000 calories or 66 pounds of potential body fat if this energy is not used as fuel for daily living.

High-carbohydrate diets that are especially high in sugar may be hazardous to one's health. They can increase the amount of triglycerides produced in the liver. These triglycerides are blood fats and are possible developers of hardened arteries. Also, a diet high in simple carbohydrates can lead to obesity, which can then result in the development of late-onset diabetes.

Alcohol is not a nutrient, but it is consumed by many people, so we will just mention it here. Like Fats and carbohydrates, it is made from carbon, oxygen and hydrogen. It holds 7 calories per gram, so you can see why it is a factor in weight control.

Alcoholic drinks are a combination of carbohydrates (4 calories per gram) and alcohol. Some, like eggnog, will also have some protein. There may be other nutrients present. There may be some B vitamins in beer and some vitamin C in screwdrivers (orange juice and vodka), mimosas (orange juice and champagne) or tropical drinks. And red wine has a healthful phytochemical called resveratrol that is a powerful antioxidant.

Caloric content of various alcoholic drinks:

Beverages	Amount	Calories
Ale,	1 bottle 12 oz	148
Beer,	1 bottle 12 oz.	173
Cider, fermented,	1 glass 8 oz.	73
Daiquiri,	1 glass 6 oz.	124
Eggnog,	1 punch cup	338
Gin, dry,	1 jigger 1.5 oz.	107
Manhattan,	1 cocktail	167
Martini,	1 cocktail	143
Whiskey, Scotch,	1 jigger 1.5 oz.	107
Wine, red,	1 wine glass	73
Wine, port,	1 glass	60

Fiber is that part of the foods we take in that is not digestible. Fiber helps to move the food through the intestines by increasing their peristaltic action. Vegetable fibers are made up chiefly of cellulose, an indigestible carbohydrate that is the main ingredient in the cell walls of plants. Plant-eating animals, such as cows, can digest cellulose. Meat-eating animals, such as humans, do not have the proper enzymes in their digestive tracts to metabolize cellulose.

Bran (which includes the husks of wheat, oats, rice, rye, and corn) is another type of fiber. It is indigestible because of the silica in the outer husks. Some of the fibers, such as wheat bran, are insoluble. Their major function is to add bulk to the feces and to speed the digested foods through the intestines. This reduces one's risk of constipation, intestinal cancer, appendicitis, and diverticulosis.

Diverticulosis is an intestinal problem that is becoming relatively frequent. It is now one of the most common intestinal disorders in Western nations. The diverticulae are pouches similar to small hernias in the intestinal wall. They are caused by either a fold of muscle in the interior wall that pushes outward, or by a weakness in the internal muscle itself. In either case, the pouch may fill with fecal matter and become infected, resulting in diverticulitis. Experts now believe that these pouches are the final stages of a long-term lack of dietary fiber.

Some types of fibers are soluble; that is, they can pick up certain substances such as dietary cholesterol. Pectin, commonly found in raw fruits (especially apple skins), oat and rice brans, and some gums from the seeds and stems of tropical plants (such as guar and xanthin) are examples of soluble fibers. These pick up cholesterols as they move through the intestines.

Foods high in fiber are also valuable in weight-reducing diets because they speed the passage of foods through the digestive tract, thereby cutting the amount of possible absorption time. They also cut the amount of hunger experienced by a dieter because they fill the stomach. A larger salad with a diet dressing might give the person very few calories but still enough cellulose to fill the stomach, cut the hunger, and move other foods through the intestinal passage.

Food processing often removes the natural fiber from the food. This is one of the primary reasons that we have relatively low amounts of fiber in our diet. For instance, white bread has only a trace of fiber -- about 9 grams in a loaf -- while old-fashioned whole wheat bread has 70 grams. Also, when you peel a carrot or an apple, you remove much of the fiber.

Dietitians urge that people include more fiber in their diets. People should be particularly conscious of the benefits of whole-grain cereals, bran and fibrous vegetables. Root vegetables (carrots, beets and turnips) and leafy vegetables are very good sources of fiber. The average diet has between 10-20 grams of fiber in it per day but recommendations to reduce colon cancer risk are between 25 and 35 grams of fiber per day.

END NOTES

1. Tarnopolsky, M. A., Atkinson, S. A., MacDougall, J. D., Chesley, A., Phillips, S., and Schwarcz, H. P. (1992). Evaluation of protein requirements for trained strength athletes. Journal of Applied Physiology, 73, 1986-95.

2. Lemon, P. W., Tarnopolsky, M. A., MacDougall, J. D., and Atkinson, S. A. (1992). Protein requirements and muscle mass/strength changes during intensive training in novice bodybuilders. Journal of Applied Physiology, 73, 767-75.

3. FAO/WHO: Energy and Protein Requirements, FAO Nutrition Report No. 52; Who Tech. Report No. 522. Rome and Geneva, 1973; FAO/WHO: Amino Acid Content of Foods and Biological Data on Proteins. No. 24. Rome, 1970.

4. Colomer R, Moreno-Nogueira JM, García-Luna PP et al. (May 2007). "N-3 fatty acids, cancer and cachexia: a systematic review of the literature". *Br. J. Nutr.* **97** (5): 823–31.

5. Evangelos C. Rizos, MD, PhD; Evangelia E. Ntzani, MD, PhD; Eftychia Bika, MD; Michael S. Kostapanos, MD; Moses S. Elisaf, MD, PhD, FASA, FRSH (September 2012). "Association Between Omega-3 Fatty Acid Supplementation and Risk of Major Cardiovascular Disease Events A Systematic Review and Meta-analysis". *JAMA* **308** (10): 1024;1033.

6. Clark, R. et al. "Dietary lipids and blood." Brit. Med. Jour. Jan. 1997, 314, p. 112)

7. Lichtenstein, Ausman, Carrasco, Jenner, Ordovas, and Schaefer, 1993).

8. Blankenhorn, D. H., and Hodis, H. N. (1993). Atherosclerosis--reversal with therapy. Western Journal of Medicine, 159, 172-9.

REFERENCE

Pennington, Jean, Church, Helen. Food Values of Portions Commonly Used. New York: Harper & Row. 2005.

(This is an essential for anyone seriously interested in nutrition. It lists nearly every food and notes protein, fat and carbohydrate contents, 10 vitamins and 9 minerals, as well as many other specialized lists of nutrients.)

CHAPTER 7
VITAMINS AND MINERALS

Vitamins are organic compounds that are essential in small amounts for the growth and development of animals and humans. They act as enzymes (catalysts) which facilitate many of the body processes to occur. Although there is great controversy as to the importance of consuming excess vitamins, it is acknowledged that we need a minimum amount of vitamins for proper functioning.

Some vitamins are soluble only in water; others need fat to be absorbed by the body. The water-soluble vitamins, B complex and C, are more fragile than the fat-soluble vitamins. This is because they are more easily destroyed by the heat of cooking and if boiled, they lose some of their potency into the water. Since they are not stored by the body, they should be included in the daily diet.

The fat-soluble vitamins, A, D, E, and K, need oils in the intestines to be absorbed by the body. They are more stable than the water-soluble vitamins and are not destroyed by normal cooking methods. Because they are stored in the body, there is the possibility of ingesting too much of them -- especially vitamins A and D.

Nutritional researchers disagree as to whether vitamin supplements are necessary. But they are generally in agreement that natural vitamins are no better than synthetically prepared vitamins. Thus, synthetically-made ascorbic acid is vitamin C. There is therefore no need to take rose hips or acerola types of the vitamin in order to get the full effect of vitamin C.

Vitamin A is necessary for eyesight as well as for skin. During World War II, Denmark began exporting large amounts of butter while supplementing Danish diets with margarine. Many children went blind. It was eventually discovered that the lack of vitamin A in the margarine was responsible for the eye problems. The minimum vitamin A requirements, which the Danes had been consuming when they were eating butter, were reduced when they substituted margarine. Vitamin A was then added to the margarine and no further problems developed.

It is possible to get too much vitamin A. When this happens the liver can enlarge. There can be a loss of appetite or weight, loss of hair, severe bone and joint pain, and cracking lips. It probably requires 20 times the minimum daily requirement over a long period of time before this would occur. A vitamin A overdose case was reported by the Food and Drug Administration when a woman had taken 75, 000 units daily for two years. Among the symptoms she had developed were hair loss, mouth ulcers, extreme fatigue, anemia, inflammation of the optic nerve, and a buildup of pressure within the head that showed the same symptoms as a brain tumor. Recently, a man died from an overdose of vitamin A over a long period of time. For this reason, the United States Food and Drug Administration has required limiting vitamin A to 10, 000 international units in any non-prescription pill.

Beta carotene is the plant source from which our bodies make vitamin A. Beta carotene does not seem to have the toxicity that vitamin A from animal sources has. Beta carotene is a powerful anti-oxidant. Along with other anti-oxidants, including vitamins C and E, and the mineral selenium, beta carotene "donates" electrons to free oxygen radicals making them less destructive.

Free oxygen radicals are harmful substances. They are atoms of oxygen which lack one electron. This makes them unstable. They therefore seek available electrons in other molecules or cells and cause damage to tissues or they can interfere with the proper chemical reactions in the body. They are believed to be associated with aging and with about sixty diseases including heart disease, cancers, arthritis, Alzheimer's disease—and even shin splints. They are also suspected of being one of the substances that can start the lesions which develop into atherosclerosis.

They are produced by many natural body processes. Physical exercise, for all of its benefits, is one producer of free oxygen radicals. They are also found in the environment. Air and water pollution, any type of smoke, and even dried milk and eggs are some of the environmental sources of these toxins.

Supplementation with anti-oxidants above required levels does not appear to increase one's aerobic capacity; however, a deficiency of vitamin C and/or vitamin E has been shown to decrease one's endurance capacity. In addition, the supplementation of anti-oxidants does not appear to prevent oxidative injury to cells during exercise, but it does appear to help decrease oxidative injury both at rest and after exercise .

In animal and human experiments relating to the effect of the anti-oxidant properties of vitamins C and E against air pollution and smoke, it was found that vitamin C is more effective in protecting against nitrogen dioxide, while vitamin E is more effective against ozone's oxidative effects. It should be noted, though, that for maximal protection against the harmful effects of air pollutants, the recommended dietary allowances for both of these vitamins should be increased. (1) Supplementation will be covered in another chapter.

The B-complex vitamins include at least 15 substances; only six have been termed essential. The B vitamins seem to work together, particularly in the nervous, circulatory, and digestive systems. Some of the B vitamins assist in the breakdown of proteins while others assist in the breakdown of carbohydrates.

Vitamin B1 (thiamin) has been linked with various theories. There is a theory of a possible link between a thiamin deficiency and Alzheimer's, but so far the data is inconclusive. Those with abnormally high intakes of alcohol, including those with cirrhosis of the liver, tend to be deficient in thiamin. However, thiamin deficiency can be reversed with supplementation. In a study on elderly people who were initially thiamin-deficient, a thiamin supplement was shown to increase appetite, energy intake, activity, body weight, and general well-being. In addition, they also showed improved sleep patterns along with reduced sleep requirements during the daytime. (2) There is some evidence that thiamin in doses of over 5 milligrams a day may act as an insect repellent since the excess of the vitamin gives the skin an odor that repels some bugs, including mosquitoes.

Vitamin B2 (riboflavin) and vitamin B6 (pyridoxine) deficiencies may prove to hamper one's fitness performance. However, if one is not deficient, there appears to be no additional fitness benefit from further supplementation of these vitamins. With an increase in exercise training, riboflavin requirements have been shown to increase] so it may be important to increase your intake of riboflavin when embarking on or increasing an existing exercise program. Also, elevated riboflavin levels may provide protection against oxidative damage. (3)

Vitamin B3 (niacin) has been found to inhibit the growth rate of some cancer cells in rats. Pellagra, a niacin deficiency disease, can lead to the development of symptoms of mental illness, such as hallucinations.

Recent research has found that when the body is high in a compound called homocysteine there is an increased chance of heart attack. Both folic acid (recommended amounts from 180 to 400 mcg per day) and vitamin B6 (recommended amount 3 mg. per day) can reduce the risk significantly. (4)

Vegans, those who consume no animal products or by-products, have diets that are usually deficient in vitamin B12. This is a concern because a vitamin B12 deficiency, in extreme cases, can cause a loss of brain function. Also, a group of vegans in England suffered irreversible destruction of nerve fibers in the spinal cord after 10 to 15 years because of their chronic vitamin B12 deficiency.

Cooking and light can destroy some of the B vitamins. Riboflavin is destroyed very quickly by light and up to 30 percent may be destroyed in cooking. Milk in a clear bottle, left in the sunlight for two hours, can lose up to 6 percent of its riboflavin. Thiamin is also destroyed by cooking, especially boiling.

Excessive B vitamins can affect the efficiency of drugs being taken, so it is important to consider where your diet is in terms of your B vitamins when taking prescription drugs. For example, riboflavin can interfere with the effects of tetracycline, an antibiotic. Pyridoxine can interfere with levadopa, which is often prescribed for Parkinson's disease. And folic acid can lessen the effects of an anti-epileptic drug.

Vitamin C is probably the most controversial of all the vitamins, largely because of Linus Pauling's publicity. Vitamin C is claimed by some to have power to cure sore backs, prevent colds, and extend life. These claims are still open to question. One of the greatest advantages of vitamin C is its antioxidant potential. In a Finnish study reported in the British Medical Journal it was found that men low in vitamin C had a far higher risk of dying from a heart attack than those with normal amounts of the vitamin. (5)

We know that people do need some vitamin C because without 10 milligrams a day, a person would get scurvy—a disease causing weakness and bleeding. In years past, before the effects of vitamin C were known, whole armies were decimated by scurvy. It is estimated that over 10,000 seamen died in the early days of sea exploration because they didn't have enough of this vitamin. However, once fresh citrus fruits were added to their diets, scurvy ceased to be a problem.

Vitamin C is made from glucose, a simple sugar found in ordinary table sugar. In order to turn the glucose into vitamin C, a special liver enzyme is required. Humans do not have that enzyme in their systems, requiring them to take in vitamin C from an outside source, such as oranges. Most other animals do have the ability to convert sugar into this necessary vitamin.

Most of the research relating to vitamin C has dealt with whether or not it can cure or prevent the common cold. Since there are at least 113 distinct viruses known to be able to cause a cold, it is unlikely that any one vitamin could work to limit all the viruses. However it does seem to have some positive effects in protecting against colds. This may be due to the effects of collagen building. Collagen is the substance essential to many body tissues, such as bone, blood vessel walls, and nearly every other tissue in the body.

Another aspect of excessive vitamin C ingestion is its possible link with anemia. A study by the National Institute of Arthritis, Metabolism, and Digestive Diseases found that large amounts of vitamin C destroy the vitamin B12 contained in food. So a daily ingestion of half a gram or more of vitamin C may result in anemia in some people.

One particular group of people may require more vitamin C than the rest of the population: smokers. This may not seem surprising in light of the earlier discussion of the protective effects of vitamin C as an anti-oxidant. It has been shown that smokers have lower blood levels of vitamin C than do non-smokers (6), and smokers with a vitamin C deficiency have a greater chance of developing certain oral mucosal lesions than do others in the population (7)

Vitamin D is seldom found to be deficient in the Western diet. New research, however, is finding that our earlier recommendation for minimum requirements was too low. It has therefore been increased from 400 IU per day to 600 IU, with those over 70 years old requiring 800 IU per day. But many researchers think that these levels are also too low, so they will probably be raised again soon.

Vitamin D can be developed by the action of ultraviolet rays from the sun on some cholesterols in the skin. Ten to twenty minutes in the sun two or three days a week should give one an entire week's supply. In fact staying in the sun until the skin is pink can generate as much as 20,000 IUs of D. However, people with darker skin and older people cannot generate as much vitamin D from sunlight as can younger lighter skinned people.

A lack of vitamin D in adults may reduce some cancers. Taking the vitamin early in life seemed to reduce the risk of breast cancer 20 years later. Prostate cancer and high blood pressure are also increased when the level of vitamin D is low. There also seems to be some relationship to depression with low blood levels of vitamin D.

Some years ago it was estimated the 1000 IU was a recommended top level for a daily dose. It is now thought to be 10,000 IU, but recommendations for ingested vitamin D is commonly at the 4000 IU level. However vitamin D generated from being in the sun seems to have no maximum.

Vitamin E, like vitamin C, has many advocates who claim unproven benefits from its use. For example, vitamin E may be able to help cells live longer. This does not mean that vitamin E will slow the aging process, but it may indicate that the vitamin can be a shield to certain environmental stresses, such as smog, radiation, and other pollutants. This is because of its anti-oxidant properties. When cells treated with vitamin E were exposed to such environmental stresses, only 30 percent stopped reproducing compared to 90 percent of the untreated cells. Other studies done at the University of Southern California have indicated that vitamin E may help to prevent emphysema and offer protection from smog by protecting both the lung tissue cells and the red blood cells as they pass through the lungs.

For over 25 years it has been recognized that the heart is benefited by adequate amounts of vitamin E. Now there is also evidence that it increases endurance (stamina) especially in those who are not well conditioned. It has also been found to reduce muscular injuries because of its anti-oxidant properties.

MINERALS

Minerals are usually structural components of the body, but they sometimes participate in certain body processes. The body uses many minerals -- phosphorus, calcium, and magnesium for strong teeth and bones; zinc for growth; chromium for carbohydrate metabolism; and copper and iron for hemoglobin production.

Iron is used primarily in developing hemoglobin, which carries the oxygen in the red blood cells. Women need more iron than men until they go through menopause (18 milligrams a day), at which time their iron requirements drop to that of men (10 milligrams a day). Iron deficiency, common in women athletes, may impair athletic performance and should be corrected with supplementation.

In the West, iron toxicity (an excess of iron) is rare. But the Bantu tribe of Africa experiences iron toxicity. This is because they cook in iron utensils and they brew their alcohol in iron, thereby greatly increasing their iron intake. There is some recent, yet still controversial, evidence that an excess of iron may increase the risk of heart disease.

Magnesium is the eighth most abundant element on the earth's surface and the fourth most abundant mineral in the body. It seems to help activate enzymes essential to energy transfer so is important in strength and endurance activities. When it is not present in sufficient amounts, twitching, tremors, and undue anxiety may develop. There is some evidence to indicate that people who are exercising should have an increased amount of magnesium.

Calcium is primarily responsible for the building of strong bones and teeth. For this, it seems obvious that a diet that is chronically low in calcium would have a negative effect on one's bone strength. The result of this is brittle and porous bones as one gets older, a condition known as osteoporosis. This is diagnosed when the bone density shows a loss of 40 percent of the necessary calcium. It happens quite often in older people, especially post-menopausal women (including surgical menopausal women), as estrogen seems to serve a protective function against bone loss. In addition, post-menopausal women exposed to excess thyroid hormone are at a greater risk for developing osteoporosis due to the increased loss of bone density seen in this population. (8) In fact, osteoporosis affects 25 percent of women and 13 percent of men over the age of 65.

The inclusion of adequate calcium (which may be higher than the current RDA) in teenage and young adult years can aid in the development of peak bone mass, which can help prevent osteoporosis later on in life. Another contributing factor to osteoporosis is the imbalance of phosphorus to calcium in the Western diet. Calcium and phosphorous work together. They should be consumed in a 1 to 1 ratio. However, the typical diet is much

49

higher in phosphorus than calcium, leading to a leeching of calcium from the bones to make up for this imbalance.

Calcium is also necessary for strong teeth, nerve transmissions, blood clotting, and muscle contractions. Without enough calcium, muscle cramps often result. It has been predicted that we will experience a great increase in gum disease in addition to weak bones because of our dietary increase in phosphorus over the last three to four decades.

Fluoride deficiency may be a primary nutritional deficiency in many parts of the Western world. It is a major cause of cavities and dental caries. Fluoride helps build stronger bones and teeth. The average citizen has 10.2 cavities. However, in Colorado Springs, where the water registers two parts per million of fluorides, the cavity rate is 0.61. In Newburgh, New York, dental caries rates were reduced by 60 percent after adding one quart per million of fluoride to the drinking water.

Potassium is a chief mineral in cell growth. A deficiency can cause impaired nerve and muscle functions ranging from paralysis to minor weakness, loss of appetite, nausea, depression, apathy, drowsiness, confusion, heart failure, and even death.

Studies have shown an increase in blood pressure when sodium intake is high. Such studies have also shown blood pressure is decreased when the potassium intake is increased. A 1 to 1 ratio of sodium to potassium is considered good—although our foraging ancestors, who did not add table salt to their foods, may have been getting 10 times as much potassium as sodium. Most people are much higher than desirable in sodium intake and lower than desirable in potassium intake.

Copper helps in the production of red blood cells. It also helps in the metabolism of glucose (sugar), with the release of energy, in the formation of fats in the nerve walls, and in the formation of connective tissues. Deficiency of copper is very rare.

Manganese is used in fat and carbohydrate metabolism, pancreas development, prevention of bone defects, muscle contraction, and many other functions. It has not yet been observed as a human deficiency.

Zinc is an ingredient in insulin and is used in carbohydrate metabolism which is necessary for energy. It is also essential in protein metabolism so is necessary for the normal growth of general organs, the prevention of anemia, and the growth of all tissues. It also helps in wound healing. It is seldom found deficient in Western Europe or the U.S. but it has been observed deficient in some people in the Middle East. People on low calorie diets may also be low in this mineral. Zinc in excess of the RDA interferes with copper absorption and decreases the level of HDL cholesterol (the "good" cholesterol) in the blood. The RDA for zinc is 12 mg per day for women and 15 mg for men.

Chromium is an essential mineral that you need in small amounts to maintain normal blood sugar balance. Both men and women need about 120 micrograms per day. If you have diabetes and are deficient in chromium, supplementation may help you control your blood sugar. Although chromium deficiency is not the primary cause of diabetes in the West, if you have a family history of late-onset (type II) diabetes, you should eat chromium-rich foods such as whole grain breads, nuts, prunes, molasses, cheese, and oysters, or consider taking a daily tablespoon of brewer's yeast.

Some people believe that it helps to build muscle and to burn fat, but there is no scientific evidence for either belief.

Selenium is a powerful antioxidant that works with vitamin E. The RDA for selenium is 55 micrograms for women and 70 micrograms for men. It is unclear whether extra selenium is helpful in reducing the risk of cell damage among heavy exercisers. Because intakes greater than 200 micrograms may be toxic, the best advice to date is to limit selenium intake to the RDA. Good food sources are meat, eggs, milk, seafood, and--depending on the amount of selenium found in soil--broccoli, garlic, mushrooms, and whole grain cereals.

Trace minerals are those that are found in very small amounts. Nearly every element found in the body is "essential," but the trace minerals are required in such small amounts and are generally abundantly found in the diet, so there is little reason for dietary deficiency. Usually foods high in calcium and iron are high in the other necessary trace minerals.

Some athletes and heavy exercisers believe that they need high doses of minerals to counter the stress of hard training. But most studies show that, except for iron (particularly among female athletes), the mineral status of highly trained athletes is similar to that of healthy, untrained people and that training does not deplete mineral status.

PHYTOCHEMICALS

Phyto (Greek for "plant") chemicals include thousands of chemical compounds which are found in plants. Some of these are vitamins and many have no known effect on us, however more and more are being found to be highly beneficial.

In the past, the phytonutrients found in fruits and vegetables were classified as vitamins: Flavonoids were known as vitamin P, cabbage factors (glucosinolates and indoles) were called vitamin U, and ubiquinone was vitamin Q. Tocopherol somehow stayed on the list as vitamin E. Vitamin designation was dropped for the other nutrients because specific deficiency symptoms could not be established and "vita" means "life" so if the compound could not be found to be absolutely essential for life it was dropped as a "vitamin" but is now classified as a phytochemical.

Various phytochemicals have been found to reduce the chance of cancers developing, reduce the chance of heart attack, reduce blood pressure and increase immunity factors. Few of these have been reduced to pill form, such as vitamin pills, so they must be consumed in fruits and vegetables daily. It is suggested that each of us consume at least five servings of raw fruits or vegetables daily. Since many of the phytochemicals are heat sensitive, cooking can destroy some or all of the active ingredients.

We are a long way from developing highly effective phytochemical supplements because there are so many elements and they may be destroyed in the processing. Garlic pills, for example, are available. However for those which have been deodorized some of the active ingredients have been removed—they were in the chemicals which gave the garlic its "aroma."

Several types of phytochemicals are being studied:

Plant sterols are somewhat similar to the animal sterol cholesterol but are unsaturated. These plant sterols compete for the same sites and thereby lower the blood cholesterol levels, often by 10%. Soy is a good source for such sterols. Most green and yellow vegetables, and particularly their seeds, contain essential sterols.

Phenols have the ability to block specific enzymes which cause inflammation. They also modify the prostaglandin pathways and thereby protect blood platelets from clumping thereby reducing the risk of blood clots. Blue, blue-red and violet colorations seen in berries, grapes and purple eggplant are due to their phenolic content. Resveratrol in red wine is a phenol.

Flavonoids is the name for a large group of compounds. They are found primarily in tea, citrus fruits, onions, soy and wine. Some can be irritating but others seem to reduce heart attack risk. For example, the phenolic substances in red wine inhibit oxidation of human LDL. The biologic activities of flavonoids include action against allergies, inflammation, free radicals, liver toxins, blood clotting, ulcers, viruses and tumors.

Terpenes such as those found in green foods, soy products and grains, comprise one of the largest classes of phytonutrients. The most intensely studied terpenes are carotenoids—as evidenced by the many recent studies on beta carotene. Only a few of the carotenoids have the antioxidant properties of beta carotene. These substances are found in bright yellow, orange and red plant pigments found in vegetables such as tomatoes, parsley, oranges, pink grapefruit, and spinach.

Limonoids are a subclass of terpenes which are found in citrus fruit peels. They appear to protect lung tissue and aid in detoxifying harmful chemicals in the liver.

Recent research is confirming suspicions of the effects of soy products and related foods which have long been used in the Oriental diets. The observation that Oriental women did not experience the problems of menopause that Western women commonly endure, such as hot flashes had long been known but no theories had yet been developed. Now we realize that a major factor is the fact that the Asians eat more vegetables, particularly soy beans.

It is the phytoestrogens, plant chemicals that mimic the effects of the female hormone estrogen, which seems to be the major factor. These plant-like estrogens have similar effects to the natural estrogen in reducing heart disease, maintaining brain functions, reducing the incidence of breast cancers, and reducing the softening of the bones (osteoporosis). Additionally other positive effects, which may or may not be related to estrogen intake, also occur, such as: reductions in cancers (prostate, endometrial, bowel) and the effects of alcohol abuse. (9)

WATER

Water is called the essential non-nutrient because it brings with it no nutritional value and yet, without it, we would die. Water makes up approximately 60 percent of the adult body, while an infant's body is nearly 80 percent water. Water is used to cool the body through perspiration, to carry nutrients to and waste products from the cells, to help cushion our vital organs, and in the makeup of all body fluids.

The body has about 18 square feet of skin that contains about 2 million sweat glands. On a comfortable day, a person will perspire about a half pint of water. Somebody exercising on a severely hot day may lose as much as 7 quarts or liters of water. This needs to be replaced or severe dehydration can result. It is therefore generally recommended that each person drink eight, 8 oz. (500 deciliters) glasses of water, or its equivalent in other fluids, daily. This amount is dependent on the climate in which you live, the altitude at which you live, the type of foods that you eat, and the amount of activity that you participate in on a day to day basis.

End Notes

--Menzel, D. B. (1992). Antioxidant vitamins and prevention of lung disease. Annals of the New York Academy of Science, 669, 141-55.

Smidt, L. J., Cremin, F. M., Grivetti, L. E., and Clifford, A. J. (1991). Influence of thiamin supplementation on the health and general well-being of an elderly Irish population with marginal thiamin deficiency. Journal of Gerontology, 46, M16-22.

Christensen, H. N. (1993). Riboflavin can protect tissue from oxidative injury. Nutritional Review, 51, 149-50.

McCully, K.S. "Homocysteine, folate, vitamin B6 and cardiovascular disease." Journal of the American Medical Association, 279, 1998, pp. 392-393; Rimm, E.B. et al. "Folate and vitamin B6 from diet and supplements in relation to risk of coronary heart disease in women." JAMA 279, 1998. Pp. 359-364.

Salonen, R. et al. "Vitamin C deficiency and risk of myocardial infarction: prospective population study of men from eastern Finland." British Med. Jour. March 1997, 314 p. 634.

Schectman, G. (1993). Estimating ascorbic acid requirements for cigarette smokers. Annals of New York Academy of Science, 686, 335-46.

Tuovinen, V., Vaananen, M., Kullaa, A., Karinpaa, A., Markkanen, H. and Kumpusalo, E. (1992). Oral mucosal changes related to plasma ascorbic acid levels. Proclaimations of the Finnish Dental Society, 88(3-4), 117-22.

Campos, P. M. M., Munoz, T. M., Escobar, J. F., Ruiz de Almodovar, M., and Jodar, G. E. (1993). Bone mass in females with different thyroid disorders: influence of menopausal status. Bone Minerals, 21, 1-8.

Bingham, S.A. et al "Phyto-oestrogens: where are we now?" Brit. J of Nutrition May, 1998, 79(5) 393-406; Willard, S.T. and Frawley, L.S. ""Phytoestrogens have agonistic and combinatorial effects on estrogen-responsive gene expression in MCF-7 human breast cancer cells," Endocrinology, Apr. 1998, 8(2), 117-121); Clarkson, T.B. "The potential of soybean phytoestrogens for postmenopausal hormone replacement therapy," Proc. Soc. Exp. Biol. Med. Mar. 1998, 217(3) 365-368.

--Blass, J. P., Sheu, K. F., Cooper, A. J., Jung, E. H., and Gibson, G. E. (1992). Thiamin and Alzheimer's disease. Journal of Nutritional Science and Vitaminology, Tokyo, Spec. No., 401-4.

Do I get enough vitamin C?
Do I get enough selenium?
Do I get too much iron?
Do I get enough vitamin D?
How can I strengthen my immune system?
Let's look and see!

Contrary to some opinions, some pills may help you live longer and better. Vitamin and mineral supplements are often helpful, especially those which include the antioxidants. Aspirin is also a major health helper with only a few side effects.

Too much of anything can cause problems. We need to look at the minimum amount of a substance which is needed, the ideal amount, and the harmful amount. For example, the minimal amount of vitamin C required to prevent the bleeding disease called "scurvy" is 10 milligrams a day. The minimum daily requirement generally listed as 30 to 50 milligrams a day. If the antioxidant properties of vitamin C are important even more of the vitamin may be desirable. Dr. Ken Cooper, the man who coined the phrase "aerobics" and began the fitness revolution in the 1960's recommends 1,000 mg. per day. (1) And some scientists have taken more than 2000 mg (2 grams) a day without ill effects. But some people have developed kidney stones from one of the binding elements used in making a vitamin C pill. Had they had enough water in their diet there would have been no problems.

Aspirin is useful in combating head and body pains and fever. It also is useful in reducing the pain of arthritis. But the major use of the drug today in the United States is to reduce the chances of having a heart attack by making the blood platelets more slippery so that they don't clump together and become blood clots or embolisms. A baby aspirin or a half of a normal aspirin is sufficient to have this desired effect.

Aspirin also has been found to reduce the incidence of skin cancers by about 15% and colon, lung and prostate cancer by as much as 46%. The risk of death dropped to a level between 15% and 37%.

It may slow the onset of Alzheimer's disease. Two of the factors related to dementia and Alzheimer's are inflammation and poor blood flow. Aspirin may reduce these. (2) It may reduce the toxicity of the typical amyloid plaques formed in Alzheimer's. (3) It is certainly not proven. (4)

Studies of aspirin however are somewhat in conflict. It should also be noted that since one of the effects of aspirin is to thin the blood, bleeding and bruising may be increased. While this reduces the likelihood of blood clots and embolisms forming, it can increase the likelihood of hemorrhaging. You remember that the causes of heart attack and stroke are most likely to be clots, embolisms and hemorrhaging. The largest danger seems to be the risk of bleeding in the stomach. It also reduces vitamin C and the B vitamin, folic acid, which is needed for DNA repair

Some people develop gastric bleeding from taking aspirin. About 4% of people are susceptible to this problem. Statistics in the United States indicate that about 17,000 people die each year from the gastric bleeding caused by aspirin and other non-steroidal anti-inflammatory drugs such as ibuprofen (Advil), acetaminophen (Tylenol), and other such compounds

For vitamin C and aspirin the plusses definitely outnumber the minuses. But how does your body tolerate such chemicals? This is the key factor. If your mother died from gastric bleeding from taking an aspirin-like compound and your father died of a heart attack, what are your odds in taking aspirin? You will undoubtedly want some

Recent evidence suggests that both heart attacks and strokes can be caused when the blood vessels are inflamed. Obviously these anti-inflammatory drugs, like aspirin, can counteract such inflammation.

Ginkgo biloba is one of the oldest, still existing plants. Extracts from its leaves were already used in ancient China whereas in the Western World, they have been utilized only since the Sixties when it became technically possible and feasible to isolate the essential substances of Ginkgo biloba. Pharmacologically, there are two groups of substances which are of some significance: the flavonoids, effective as oxygen-free radical scavengers, and the terpenes (i.e. the ginkgolides) with their highly specific action in slowing blood clot formation. (5)

Ginko bilboa seems to have the effect of stabilizing or reducing (20% of cases) the effects of dementia which often comes with old age. (6)

Among the reasons given for its potential effectiveness are that it may:

protect against brain cell damage by a chemical called glutamate which might allow excess calcium infiltration into brain cells;

--prevent a constriction of the brain's blood vessels;

--aid in keeping the blood vessels elastic.

In one study those taking the ginko bilboa, two out of three people improved in their tests measuring: attention, memory, behavior and their abilities to perform necessary activities of daily life. It seems to work not only in slowing or stopping brain deterioration but in preventing it.

MULTI-VITAMIN AND MINERAL SUPPLEMENTS

Many people do not eat a well balanced diet so they decide to supplement their diets with multiple vitamins. Based on the number of multi-vitamin pills sold, it appears that most Americans believe that their diets are deficient!

While many people take a multivitamin and possibly a multi-mineral pill daily they may not be aware that they might be getting too much of an element. For example, while most women may need extra iron, most men do not need any more than they get in their normal diet. Excessive iron may be a negative factor in heart disease.

Many people do not get enough vitamin B 12, this is particularly true of those who do not eat meat. Consequently this vitamin might be necessary to supplement. Having a complete blood analysis should be helpful for you and your doctor in developing a sensible supplement plan.

THE ANTIOXIDENT SUPPLEMENTS

As you are well aware, a free oxygen radical, that is an atom of oxygen rather than the common oxygen molecule that has two atoms--O_2. The single atom is unstable because there is room in its outer ring for two more electrons to stabilize it. In looking for stabilizing substances these free oxygen radicals can damage many parts of our bodies, especially the inner linings of our blood vessels. Antioxidant supplements provide options for the free oxygen radicals to attack and thereby save them from damaging parts of the body.

Exercise, breathing smog, and in fact just living create these free oxygen radicals. It is therefore wise to supply the body with substances that can neutralize them. Here are some such nutrients. If you decide to supplement with some of these, combinations can often be found in one pill.

BETA CAROTENE

Beta carotene is a precursor to vitamin A. If you haven't taken in sufficient vitamin A through milk, eggs, live, cheese, butter or fish oil, 6 units of beta carotene can be converted into one unit of vitamin A. What is left acts as a strong antioxidant. It can lower the risk cataracts --a clouding in the lens of the eye which blurs vision which often occurs with age. It also reduces the risk of many cancers, particularly lung, lung, bladder, rectal, and the serious skin cancer called melanoma.

There is no recommended minimum daily requirement for this substance but the vitamin A which it can make has a minimum recommended daily amount of 4,000 international units (I.U.) for women and 5,000 for men. Dr. Cooper's recommendation is 25,000 international units per day of beta carotene. (7)

VITAMIN C

Vitamin C has a minimum daily requirement (MDR) or "daily values" (DV) of 30 to 50 mg. (60 mg for smokers). It may make the cholesterol level more favorable by lowering total cholesterol but raising the good HDL (heavy density lipids). It is an antioxidant that may reduce the risk of cataracts. Some cancer risk may also be lessened (larynx, esophagus, mouth, pancreas, and stomach). In addition, by increasing immunity, it may reduce your chances of contracting infections such as a cold.

Many people have been taking 250 to 500 mg daily for years but Dr. Cooper is now recommending 1000 mg per day as a supplement. You can also get that amount by eating 13 to 17 oranges or 44 tomatoes a day. Fifteen oranges will add 1100 calories to your diet while the 40 tomatoes will add 950 calories to your daily intake. So if calories are a concern, the vitamin pill may be your better solution.

VITAMIN E

Vitamin E is a strong antioxidant which also acts as an anticoagulant—that is it reduces the blood's ability to clot so it reduces the risk of a coronary thrombus, a primary cause of heart attack, and brain embolisms, a primary cause of strokes. As the other antioxidants, it reduces the risk of some cancers, of cataracts in the lenses of the eyes, and it increases immunity to other diseases. In those who exercise Vitamin E also seems to reduce injuries to the small muscle fibers and may be important in preventing such conditions as "shin splints."

Reports in the British Medical Journal indicate that 2000 units of vitamin E delayed both the onset of Alzheimer's and the time of death. In the Cambridge Heart Antioxidant Study 400 to 800 units of vitamin E daily considerably reduced the death rate from heart disease.

Vitamin E is measured in either international units (solid form foods) or milligrams (if in oils). If measured in IU (international units) it will be about 50% higher—so 150 IU would be about 100 mg (milligrams). The minimum daily requirement for adults is only 15 milligrams (or 22.5 IU) and most people get that much in their daily diets. But for extra antioxidant protection you may want to supplement. Dr. Cooper recommends 400 units per day and many people have taken more than double that amount without any apparent risk. If you want to take your 400 I.U. in foods you can eat 300 cups of instant oat cereal (43,500 calories), 6 ½ pounds of potato chips (16,000 calories), or 32 pounds of canned tuna in oil (31,000 calories). Since 3500 calories will put on one pound of body weight for the average person you will gain between 5 and 10 pounds a day if you want to get 400 units of vitamin E through "natural" sources. And the "chemical" in the pill is the same chemical found in the oats or the tuna.

A recent study indicates another aspect of this desirable type of supplementation. Mortality from coronary heart disease in 50-54 year old men was found to be four times higher in Lithuania than in Sweden. Most risk factors were similar between the men in the two countries. The major difference seemed to be in the antioxidant intakes, particularly vitamin E. The Lithuanians were much lower. This corresponds with a study in England that showed that vitamin E supplements of from 400 to 800 IU daily reduced the death rate from heart attacks by 47%. (8)

There is also evidence that oxidative stress is involved in dementia and Alzheimer's. Work in this area may indicate that vitamin E may reduce such damage. (9) There are many more positive findings for intelligent supplementation with vitamin. There have been some cases of excess doses, but the evidence clearly indicates some level if supplementation.

COENZYME Q 10

Coenzyme Q 10 (ubiquinone) is another antioxidant. It has been linked to DNA related problems in both the nerves and the muscles. (10) It also works with both vitamin C and vitamin E in a number of actions in which all three are utilized together. (11) It also works to reduce some of the problems people may experience when taking cholesterol lowering statins.

As often happens, the research of the local scientists can influence the acceptance of the substance. While Q 10 has been studied in the United States, Dr. Cooper does not recommend it as a daily antioxidant. On the other hand, the work of Jan Karlsson and others in Sweden makes Q 10 a favorite among the Nordic peoples. The Swedish National Food Administration recommends 2 to 20 mg per day. Jan Karlsson recommends 50 to 100 mg per day with elite athletes taking in 100 to 300 mg per day. (12)

SELENIUM

Selenium is a mineral that is part of an essential enzyme (glutathione peroxidase) which protects a naturally occurring antioxidant (glutathione). It works with vitamins C, E and beta carotene. It may, as vitamin E, reduce micro-injuries to the small muscle fibers. It may also reduce the risk of digestive cancers, especially of the stomach and esophagus. In fact it seems to be protective against all cancers. (13) It is found in greater abundance in North American soils than in European soils. It therefore is found more often in both plants and animals raised in America. (14)

Side effects of an excess of selenium can include hair loss, digestive problems (vomiting, diarrhea, nausea), irritability, nerve cell problems, and fatigue. Dr. Cooper considers supplementation of selenium optional as long as you are getting 50 to 100 mg. a day. Natural sources include: 3 ½ ounces of tuna (115 mg. of selenium); a half ounce of tortilla chips (120 mg of selenium); 3 ½ ounces of lasagna noodles (96 mg.) or spaghetti (65 mg). So it is quite easy to get this mineral in a normal diet. However fruits and vegetables are quite low in selenium. But meats, grains and beans are generally high.

RESVERATROL

Resveratrol, a phytochemical found in red wine, is also found in a pill form. The pill form may contain as much resveratrol as is found in a bottle of red wine.

SOME RECOMENDATIONS

Dr. Dean Ornish's Preventive Medicine Research Institute (PMRI) conducts pioneering research on lifestyle (diet, exercise, stress management, and group support) and heart disease. Says PMRI's research director, Larry Scherwitz, PhD, If a three-day nutritional analysis reveals program participants are not obtaining adequate antioxidant levels in the diet, we recommend a range of supplementation: one to three grams vitamin C; 100 to 400 IUs of dry vitamin E daily; 10,000 to 25,000 IUs of beta

Alliance for Aging Research (AAR), based on 200 clinical studies, recommends: that people at high risk for cancer, especially asbestos workers and smokers, should not take any beta carotene supplements. For others interested in health promotion and disease prevention, they recommend the following ranges of supplements (in an aging population): vitamin C, 250 to 1000 mg daily; vitamin E, 100 to 400 IUs daily; beta carotene, 17,000 to 50,000 IUs (10 to 30 mg) daily.

The University of California Wellness Letter based on the National Cancer Institute's findings, have withdrawn their recommendation for smokers to take beta carotene supplements-though they see no harm or benefit for non-smokers to take low doses if it's not obtained in the diet. Their recommendation: In addition to eating five or more servings of fruits and vegetables daily, take 200 to 800 IUs (133 to 533 mg) of vitamin E daily; 250 to 500 mg of vitamin C, but no more than 6 to 16 mg beta carotene daily for non-smokers not obtaining adequate amounts in their diet.

OTHER CONSIDERATIONS
CALCIUM SUPPLEMENTATION

People with osteoporosis are generally required to supplement with calcium and vitamin D. Calcitonin, a nasal spray, has been found to be effective in replacing lost calcium in the bones. This is particularly true for the lumbar spine area. (15)

OMEGA 3 FATTY ACIDS

Everyone has heard of the benefits of fish oils in reducing heart disease. These essential fatty acids (EFA) were given the name of ''vitamin F'' in the 1920's. While desirable, they are no longer viewed as vitamins. These oils are part of the polyunsaturated fats (PUFA) group. Most people obtain enough of these fatty acids in their diets— particularly if they consume, fish. As mentioned earlier, fish oil capsules can supplement a lack of fish in the diet.

There are fish oil pills which can be consumed but they don't seem to be as effective as eating fish. Also, we don't know what the proper dosage of pills might be and whether there are any adverse side effects from their use. So here is one area where the ''natural'' food seems better than the pill. You should consume fish about three times a week or more. We also don't know if the benefits from eating fish come only from the oil or is there some hidden benefit from the non-oily parts of the fish. Still, fish oil supplements, from fish muscle, have been tried in a number of studies and have proven somewhat effective in reducing pain. The ideal dose seems to be 2 to 3 grams of omega 3 oil daily. (16)

It must be mentioned, however, that increasing the amount of omega 3 fatty acids requires a great intake of vitamin E because vitamin E is reduced when omega 3's are increased.

Since the omega 3 fatty acids are more easily destroyed by oxidation, the antioxidant vitamins (E, C, and beta carotene) are essential to protect them from disintegrating.

VITAMIN D

As mentioned in the chapter on vitamins, if you do not get enough sunlight you are probably low in the higher recommended levels of vitamin D.

FIBERS

Fibers are found to reduce the incidence of intestinal problems such as intestinal cancers and diverticulitis as well as blood vessel diseases, if they reduce the amount of cholesterol. Insoluble fibers such as wheat bran and silica help move food through the intestines. Soluble fibers not only move things through the intestines but also pick up cholesterols and prevent them from entering the bloodstream. It would therefore be wise for most people to take some supplements of the soluble fiber type. These include: rice bran, oat bran and apple pectin.

MELATONIN

Melatonin has been touted as a substance which can ''strengthen the body's immune system'' and is used to reduce the effects of jet lag. It seems to reduce some types of pain and to aid one's sleep. (17) Many older people take it as an aid for sleep.

DHEA

DHEA, like melatonin, is a natural hormone that reduces as we age. There is some evidence that it reduces the risk factors for heart disease. (18)

BEING A WISE CONSUMER

A number of useless products are advertised in the media. For many there is absolutely no scientific proof of their working—except for a possible placebo effect in which a person gets some benefits because he or she "thinks" the product will benefit them. When in doubt, go to the internet at "Mayo Clinic." "MedlinePlus" or "Medline" and get an idea from medical scientists.

If you are going to use some supplements, a number of health specialists, such as the previously mentioned Dr. Castelli of the Framingham study, us the low priced quality supplements sold by Puritan Pride (puritan.com). It has an extensive online and print catalogue.

Wherever you buy, note the dosage and cost. The U.S. allows for higher doses than some countries. A recent comparison of price per milligram of several supplements in Norway showed that a milligram of an element cost a hundred times more in Norway than in the US.

Supplementing your nutritional needs through vitamin or mineral pills. Buying vitamin pills should be determined by what you need. Some people need more of a vitamin than do others. For instance, if you were thinking of conceiving a child you might take some special vitamins, such as folic acid, which might decrease the chances of neural-tube defects in the baby. Some people may require a special kind of vitamin, such as a water-soluble vitamin A, for example. When restricting caloric intake for weight loss, it is a good idea to take a multivitamin and mineral supplement as it is difficult to get all the vitamins and minerals you need while on a "diet."

Labeling is often confusing. Does the label state 100 milligrams of magnesium gluconate or does it say 5.4 milligrams of magnesium? Both mean the same in terms of meeting your body's requirements for magnesium. Does it state 325 milligrams of calcium lactate or 42 milligrams of calcium? Again, they both mean the same to your body.

When you purchase supplements, try to match the voids in your diet to the vitamin pill. You might have a knowledgeable doctor or a registered dietitian analyze your diet, then get the exact dietary supplement or supplements that you need.

Most people are very low in magnesium and most pre-menopausal women are low in iron, so you may want to include these in your supplement if you find that you are deficient in these. If you don't eat citrus fruits or tomatoes, you may be low in vitamin C. If you don't eat meat or wheat, you may be low in the B vitamins. And if you don't eat whole grain cereals, you may be low in vitamin E.

Some vitamins, such as A, B_1, and C, are inexpensive to produce in the amounts needed for our daily minimal requirements. Others, such as pyridoxine, niacin, pantothenic acid or vitamin E, are expensive; consequently, many inexpensive vitamin preparations have the inexpensive vitamins without having the other vitamins. Again, be sure you know what vitamins/minerals you need and in what doses, and then check to be sure that the supplement you've chosen best suits your needs.

END NOTES

Cooper, Ken. The Antioxident Revolution. Nashville, TN: Thomas Nelson Inc., 1994, p. 119.

Casoli T, Balietti M, Giorgetti B, Solazzi M, Scarpino O, Fattoretti P. Platelets in Alzheimer's Disease-Associated Cellular Senescence and Inflammation. Curr Pharm Des. 2012 Oct 2. Neuroscience. 2011 Oct 13;193:80-8.

Liu YY, Sparatori A., Del Soldato P, Bian JS. H2S releasing aspirin protects amyloid beta induced cell toxicity in BV-2 microglial cells. Neuroscience. 2012 Sep 27;221:225.

Jaturapatporn D, Isaac MG, McCleery J, Tabet N. Aspirin, steroidal and non-steroidal anti-inflammatory drugs for the treatment of Alzheimer's disease. Cochranane Data Base 2012 Feb 15;2

Z'Brun A. "Ginkgo--myth and reality." Schweiz Rundsch Med Prax 1995 Jan 3;84(1):1-6.

Cited in British Medical Journal, Oct. 25, 1997 from: Journal of the American Medical Assn 278 1997, pp. 1327-32.

Cooper, Ibid.

Kristenson et al. Brit. Med. Jour. March 1997, 314 p. 7081.

Polidori MC, Stahl W, De Spirt S, Pientka L. Influence of vascular comorbidities on the antioxidant defense system in Alzheimer'sdisease. Dtsch Med Wochenschr. 2012 Feb;137(7):305-8.

Karlsson, J. Antioxidants and Exercise. Champaign, IL: Human Kinetics. 1997, p. 63; Halliwell, B. and Gutterudge, M. ''Oxygen free radicals and iron in relation to biology and medicine: Some problems and concepts.'' Arch. Biochem.Biophys. 246:501-514 (1986); Alessio, H.M. et al. ''Evidence that DNA damage and repair cycle activity increases following a marathon race,'' Medical Science in Sport and Exercise, 22:751 (1990); Alesio, H.M. ''Exercise-induced oxidative stress,''Med. Sci. Sports Exerc. 25:218-224, (1993)

Karlsson, J. "Advances in Nutrition for High-Intensity Training." Presentation at the World Congress of Sports Medicine, Orlando, FL, June 3, 1998.

Karlsson, J. Antioxidants and Exercise. Champaign, IL: Human Kinetics. 1997, p. 105.

Han X, Li J, Brasky TM, Xun P, Stevens J, White E, Gammon MD, He K. Antioxidant intake and pancreatic cancer risk: The Vitamins and Lifestyle (VITAL) Study. Cancer. 2012 Dec 21.

Rayman, MP "Selenium:a time to act." Brit. Medical J. 314(387) Feb. 1997,Editorial

Drinkwater, B. "Osteoporosis." Presentation at the World Congress of Sports Medicine, Orlando, FL, June 2, 1998

Karlsson, J. Op. Cit. P. 169, 170

J Vidor LP, Torres IL, de Souza IC, Fregni F, Caumo W. Analgesic and Sedative Effects of Melatonin in Temporomandibular Disorders: A Double-Blind, Randomized, Parallel-Group, Placebo-Controlled Study. Pain Symptom Management. Nov. 27, 2012.

Savineau JP, Mathan. Role of DHEA in cardiovascular diseases. Biochem Pharmacol. 2012 Dec 24.

CHAPTER 9
HEALTHY EATING

Applying our nutritional knowledge to the dinner table

The ultimate diet. Eat all the food you want. But after dessert, eat four cloves of garlic and three ounces of Limburger cheese. You don't really lose any weight, but you look thinner from a distance.

With an intelligent diet you will:
Live longer
Look better
Feel better
Here's why"

In the 1930s research showed that a reduction in food intake could greatly extend the life of monkeys in a laboratory. Since that time a number of studies from insects to animals have shown the same life extending results of a reduced calorie diet. In 2009 a 20 year study on rhesus monkeys, taking in 70% of the normal dietary calories, showed fewer AIDS-related deaths among monkeys and they were healthier as they aged. They had less diabetes, cancer, brain atrophy and cardiovascular disease. However more recently a study from the national Institute on aging indicated that while other diseases seem to be reduced, cardiovascular disease and age-related death did not seem to be affected. Part of the reason for the discrepancy in the studies may be that in the first study the control monkeys were able to eat as much as they wanted while in the second study there were not, in fact the calories were somewhat restricted. So they may have had some benefits from the reduced calorie diet. Also the control monkeys in the first study received 30% of their diet in table sugar while in the second study the control monkeys only received 4% of their diet and sugar. (1)

Sensible eating requires an understanding of the basic principles of nutrition discussed in the previous 10s. The nutrients must appear in the diet in proper quantities, and the calories must be the amount necessary in order to maintain one's desired weight. If the desired weight isn't maintained, then obesity may develop and diseases associated with obesity, such as diabetes, high blood pressure, and heart disease, can begin.

There are other factors that the sensible eater must understand. Caloric needs change according to climate and the amount of activity in which the person participates. It is obvious that hot weather necessitates a greater intake of fluids due to the loss of water through perspiration. There is also a lesser need for calories because the body does not need to burn as many calories to maintain its normal temperature.

A person using a great many calories, such as an athlete, needs more carbohydrates. It is a myth that athletes need a great deal more protein than non-athletes. While the caloric needs may nearly double for the athlete who is expending a great deal of energy, the protein needs are increased only slightly, usually less than 30 percent. Another myth concerning athletes is that they require more vitamins and minerals than do others. Supplements given to athletes already consuming well-balanced diets have not been shown to improve performance. It may well be the desire to be thin (which leads to a decrease in the nutritional quality consumed due to the decrease in caloric intake) and not the exercise training that affects the dietary practices of athletes, particularly females.(2)

Sensible eating also requires that we know how to prepare food, that we don't overspend our money on food, and that we are aware of the food fads that keep cropping up in our culture. We also need to give some thought to how we might effectively lose weight if we're overweight.

It is also important to know the effect of various foods on the teeth and on other organs, how we might prevent some of the food-borne diseases, and also how we might prevent diseases that may be caused by an improper diet.

IMPORTANT CONSIDERATIONS IN SELECTING YOUR DIET

SELF TEST

Place the appropriate number which best describes your answer to each question:
3--Almost always 2—Sometimes 1--Almost never

_____ 1. Do you eat 3 or more pieces of fruit per day? (Fruit juice counts as one piece.)

_____ 2. Do you eat a minimum of 3 servings of vegetables each day--including a green leafy or orange vegetable.)?

_____ 3. Do you eat 3 or 4 milk products per day? (such as milk, cheese, yogurt)

_____ 4. Do you eat a minimum of 6 servings of grain products each day? (breads, cereal, pasta)

_____ 5. Do you eat breakfast?

_____ 6. Do you eat fish at least three times per week?

_____ 7. Do you avoid fried foods? (including potato chips, fries)

_____ 8. Do you eat fast food four or more times per week?

_____ 9. Are the milk products you consume made from non-fat milk?

_____ 10. Do you avoid high sugar foods and highly refined carbohydrates? (such as sweet rolls, cookies, non-diet sodas, candy, etc.)

Score 25-30 You are balancing your diet well.

18-24 Your diet can use improving.

10 - 17 your diet is unhealthy.

The US Department of Agriculture's recommendations are that for most people it is recommended that they consume 6 ounces of grain, 2 ½ cups of vegetables, 2 cups of fruit, 3 cups of milk and five at half ounces of meat and beans.

To clarify, and even to improve on, the government's recommendations let us look at their suggestions.

Grain products give the carbohydrates needed for quick energy. A serving size would be one slice of bread, an ounce of dry cereal, or a half cup of cooked cereal, pasta, or rice. Daily needs range from 6 to 11 servings.

The grains are rich in B vitamins, some minerals, and fiber. They also contain some protein. Whole grains are the best sources of fibers. Refining grains or polishing rice reduces the fiber, the mineral content, and the B vitamins. This occurs in white and wheat bread (not whole wheat), pastas, pastries, and white rice. The flour is often refortified with 3 of the B complex vitamins, but seldom with the other essential nutrients.

If you are concerned with reducing your cholesterol level, thereby reducing your chances of heart disease, reducing your chances of developing gall stones, or having a softer stool in your bowel movement, eat more of the soluble fibers (oat bran cereals, whole grain bread with oats, carrots, whole potatoes, whole apples, and citrus juices that contain the pulp of the fruit, or rice bran). Many bakeries today are making interesting and healthy whole grain breads—sometimes with olives, sometimes stone ground, sometimes with multi-grain blends. There are supplements with oat bran, apple pectin and rice bran. If your concern is reducing your risk of intestinal cancers, appendicitis, and diverticulosis, eat more of the insoluble fibers (whole wheat breads and cereals, wheat bran cereals, corn cereals, prunes, beans, peas, nuts, most vegetables, and polished rice).

Vegetables contain some vitamins and minerals as well as fibers. The color of the vegetable (red, yellow, orange, green, purple, white) gives a hint as to the type of vitamins and phyto-chemicals (plant chemicals) contained in it. Among the most nutritious vegetables are: broccoli, carrots, peas, peppers, and sweet potatoes. If you are trying to lose weight many vegetables are high in water and in fibers but low in calories. Among these are all greens (lettuce, cabbage, celery) as well as cauliflower. Actually most vegetables are quite low in calories. A serving size would be a half cup of raw or cooked vegetables or a cup of raw leafy vegetables. You need 5 servings daily.

Fruits are generally high in vitamin C and fiber. They are also relatively low in calories. A serving size would be 1/4 cup of dried fruit, 1/2 cup of cooked fruit, a whole piece of fruit, or a wedge of a melon. You should have 4 servings daily. Commercial fruit juices often have added sugar so may not be particularly healthy.

A cup of raw raspberries is very high in fiber (10 gms) and antioxidants (ellagic acid and 32mg Vitamin C) and has about zero sodium and fat. But it does contain 64 calories. They could be an outstanding choice for a dessert or a snack.

Protein sources such as meats, eggs, nuts, and beans, are also high in minerals and vitamins B6 and B12. A serving would be 2 1/2 ounces of cooked meat, poultry or fish, 2 egg whites, 4 tablespoons of peanut butter, 1 1/4 cup of cooked beans. You need 2 to 3 servings a day. A McDonalds' "Quarter Pounder" would give you two servings. The hidden eggs in cakes and cookies would also count. The best meat products to eat are fish, because of the omega 3 oils which reduce blood clotting and the higher quality of protein. Egg whites have the best quality of protein. Milk is second. Of course the fat in milk is a negative so nonfat milk is better.

Muscle meats, like steak and hamburger, have a relatively low quality of protein (after egg white, milk, fish, poultry, and organ meats) and they are linked to both cancers (2 1/2 times the risk for colon cancer) and heart disease. They also carry a great amount of fat, even if the fat on the outside is trimmed off. There is also 8olesterol in the meat and fat of all land animals. Taking the skin off of poultry significantly reduces the amount of

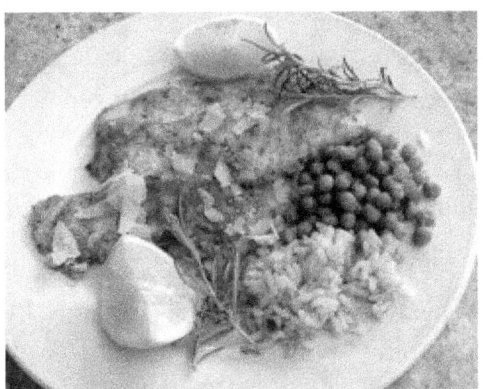

fat and cholesterol that will be consumed. Poultry carry much of their fat next to the skin.

Of the "flesh" proteins, fish is the best. It is a higher quality of protein than meat or poultry, and it contains the helpful omega 3 oils. Fish are able to convert the polyunsaturated linolenic fatty acid from plants that they eat into omega 3 oils. These work to prevent heart disease by reducing cholesterol and by making the blood less likely to clot in the arteries. They do this by interfering with the production of the hormone-like prostaglandin "thromboxane" which increases blood clotting. Clotting is therefore reduced.

Comparing steak to fish--a 3 ounce (85 gram) steak has 177 calories, 77 from fat. About 13% of its calories come from saturated fat and 16% from monounsaturated fat. It would have about 20 to 25 grams of protein. It also has 25 mg of omega 3 fat. It has no fiber but is reasonably good in the minerals. But the sodium is high. But most steak servings are 8 to 16 ounces so these figures should be multiplied by 3 to 5 to get a more accurate picture.

Three ounces of salmon would contain 140 calories, 17 grams of higher quality protein, 7.5 grams of fat of which 16% is omega 3 fats (492 mg EPA and 820 mg of DHA). It would also contain 170 IU of vitamin A and 1100 IU of vitamin D (twice the RDA) The same 3 ounces of tuna would contain 270 calories, 18 grams of protein, 20 grams of fat of which 7% is omega 3 (1100 mg of EPA and 240 mg of DHA). It also 850

IU of vitamin A (16% RDA) and 6000 IU of vitamin D—about a 10 times the RDA. So you can understand that all protein sources are not nutritionally equal.

Milk and milk products (cheeses, yogurt, ice cream) are high in calcium and protein as well as some minerals (potassium and zinc) and riboflavin. A serving would be one cup of milk or yogurt, 1 1/2 ounces of cheese, 2 cups of cottage cheese, 1 1/2 cups of ice cream, or 1 cup of pudding or custard. Adults need 2 servings daily, children need 3.

The advantage of milk products is that their protein is second only to the protein in egg whites in quality. The problem with milk products is that they usually come with saturated fats, which are of course the worst type. Whole milk gets half of its calories from the 3.5% fat in it. If you drink 2% fat milk, you have reduced the fat by 40% and the total calories by 20%. An 8 ounce glass of whole milk would have 150 calories and would contain 8 grams of fat. If it were 2% fat milk it would contain 120 calories and 4.5 grams of fat. If it were 1% fat milk it would contain 100 calories and 2.5 grams of fat. And, if we were non-fat or skim milk it would contain 80 calories. Many people think that 2% fat milk has had 98% of its fat removed, but only 40% has been removed.

People who are used to the thick taste of whole milk may find the watery consistency of skim milk unsatisfying. Just as those who are used to drinking skim milk find whole milk too thick for their tastes. So it seems that it is whenever we are used to that is the most palatable.

Cheeses vary in both fat content and calories. But an average cheese would have about 130 calories per ounce including about 90 calories of fat, of which 60 calories would be in saturated fat. There are some cheeses made from skim milk or nonfat milk that are lower in calories and fats, but they don't satisfy taste buds of many dedicated cheese aficionados.

Ice cream and custards also tend to be quite high in fats as well as in sugars. If you like cold sweet things you might be able to find frozen non-fat yogurt with artificial sweetening. Usually there are trade-offs for people who seriously want to control your weight or the quality of food that they eat.

Looking at high quality ice cream and comparing it to low fat frozen yogurt we find that in a half cup (88 grams) each has 4 grams of protein. The vanilla ice cream has 230 calories and 14 grams of fat. Chocolate chip cookie dough flavor adds 40 calories. A low fat frozen yogurt drops the calories to 130 and the fat to 3 grams. Fat free yogurt drops the calories to 105 to 120. Making the frozen yogurt fat free and sugar free drops another 25 calories—to the 80 to 95 range. So all frozen desserts are not created equal.

Fats and sweets are consumed at too high a level in the American diet. Since they have more than twice as many calories as proteins or carbohydrates this should be a real concern for people trying to control their weight. Also since they are related to a number of cancers and heart problems, they should certainly be minimized. While the average American consumes about 45% of his diet in fats, it is a concern. The government, knowing that Americans like their fat, recommends cutting to 30% with an even division between saturated, polyunsaturated and monounsaturated fats. But for those who are seriously concerned with either preventing degenerative diseases or with maintaining their weight, somewhere between the minimum 10% and 20% of total fat may be tolerable. The preferred fat type is of course the mono-unsaturates.

Butter of course is very high in saturated fats, so if you must have grease on your bread it would be best to use a soft margarine—preferably made from canola oil. A pat of butter (on inch square and a quarter inch high) contains 36 calories—all saturated fat. You might think of doing as they do in many Italian restaurants, use olive oil to wet your bread. It would be preferable to buy tasty whole-grain breads and eat them without grease.

For salad dressings canola oil or olive oil with vinegar, such as balsamic, would give you the healthiest type of fat. If you are trying to control calories use a no fat dressing. But check for the type of thickeners that are used to replace the oil. Most use a guar gum or a xanthin gum. Both are soluble fibers so they take cholesterol from the intestines while not adding any fat or cholesterol to your intake. So most nonfat salad dressings are much healthier than is generally known.

Never fry foods in oil, use a non-stick pan. If you must have an oil use canola, olive, or safflower oil. Stay away from all fried foods, including potato chips. Fried foods not only add calories and saturated fats but they increase one's chances for intestinal cancers-- as do all fats.

Sweets may assist in the development of tooth caries (cavities) but are not otherwise harmful if calories are not a problem for you. An athlete consuming 5,000 calories in a day can probably eat candy bars and ice cream, the person attempting to control one's weight should avoid them.

BEVERAGES

Beverages make up a large part of our diet. We often don't think too much about the kinds of liquids we drink. The most nutritious drinks have been rated by Michael Jacobson, co-director of the Center for Science in the Public Interest. He rated them according to the amount of fat and sugar (higher content = lower rating), and their amount of protein, vitamins, and minerals (higher content = higher rating). His results were that skim or nonfat milk was rated a +47, whole milk +38 (the lower rating was because of its fat content), orange juice +33, Hi-C +4, coffee 0, coffee with cream -1, coffee with sugar -12, Kool-Aid -55, and soft drinks -92.

Non-fat milk is the best beverage for most people. Children should have three to four cups each day. Adults should drink two cups. Our need for milk can be satisfied by other dairy products. For example, two cups of milk are equivalent to three cups of cottage cheese or five large scoops of ice cream (of course, this choice may taste the best, but there are obvious drawbacks to eating five scoops of ice cream everyday!). In addition to its nutrient value as a developer of bones and organs, milk has been found to help people sleep. They go to sleep quicker, then sleep longer and sounder. This is because of the high content of the amino acid tryptophan which makes serotonin, the neurotransmitter associated with relaxation and calming activity.

Coffee contains several ingredients that may be harmful to the body. There are stimulants such as caffeine and the xanthines. There are oils that seem to stimulate the secretion of excess acid in the stomach. And there are diuretics that eliminate water and some nutrients, such as calcium, from the body. Even two cups a day increases the risk of bone fractures. (3) A factor that may add to the risk of bone fractures is that people who drink more coffee usually drink little or no milk.

Caffeine is found in coffee, tea, and cola drinks. Brewed coffee contains 100 to 150 milligrams of caffeine per cup (mg/cup), instant coffee about 90 mg/cup, tea between 45 and 75 mg/cup, and cola drinks from 40 to 60 mg/cup. Decaffeinated coffee is virtually free of caffeine, as it contains only 2 to 4 milligrams per cup. The therapeutic dose of caffeine given to people who have overdosed on barbiturates is 43 milligrams. Yet a cup of coffee contains up to 150 milligrams of caffeine!

Caffeine is a central nervous system stimulant. It elevates one's blood pressure and constricts the blood vessels. Both of these may assist in the development of high blood pressure. It has also been reported that excess caffeine in coffee, tea, and cola drinks can produce the same symptoms found in someone suffering from psychological anxiety. These symptoms include the following: nervousness, irritability, occasional muscle twitching, sensory disturbances, diarrhea, insomnia, irregular heart beat, a drop in blood pressure, and occasionally failures of the blood circulation system.

Coffee has been a subject of controversy as a beverage for the last several years. The amount of coffee being drunk in the United States has been decreasing somewhat since its 1962 peak when people averaged over three cups a day. It is now down to just over two cups a day per person. Conflicting studies have reported that coffee is and is not a causative agent in heart disease based on its ability to increase one's blood pressure.

However, if someone already has a heart problem, it may be wise to give up coffee. This is especially true if the person ingests five cups or more a day, since it can damage the central nervous system and elevate the amount of fatty acids and sugar found in the blood. For some reason decaffeinated coffee, in large amounts, increases the risk of heart disease.

Coffee is an irritant. The oils in coffee irritate the lining of the stomach and the upper intestines. People who drink two or more cups of coffee per day increase their chances of getting ulcers by 72 percent over non-coffee drinkers. Decaffeinated coffee is no more soothing to the ulcer patient than the regular blend, because both types increase the acid secretions in the stomach. Since an ulcer patient's acid secretion is not as high when caffeine alone is ingested (when compared to the acid levels after the ingestion of decaffeinated coffee), some other ingredient in coffee is thought to be responsible for these increasing stomach acid levels.

It is best not to start children drinking coffee. And it may be better for you to decrease your own caffeine habit. If you think you need a cup of coffee in the morning to get started, switch to decaffeinated coffee and see how you feel. If you still think you need the caffeine to get going, you can try drinking some cold coffee and see if that makes you feel ready to face your day. Some people who are addicted to caffeine find that they suffer from headaches when they do not have their caffeine. If you are one of these people, you may decide to slowly decrease your caffeine intake over time to allow your body the time it needs to readjust to lower caffeine levels.

Tea is not as irritating as coffee, but it does contain some caffeine and tannic acid, which can irritate the stomach. If you drink large amounts of tea, you should take it either with milk to neutralize the acid or add ice to dilute it. Green tea, the type drunk commonly in the Orient, contains polyphenols that appear to be anti-oxidants which may reduce cancer incidence. The black tea, drunk commonly in Europe and America, has less of these protective substances. (4) Not much is known about the effects of herbal teas.

Alcohol. There are seven calories in a gram of alcohol. These calories contain no nutritional elements, but they do contribute to your total caloric intake. Since alcoholic drinks are surprisingly high in calories, they greatly contribute to the overweight problems of many individuals. People who drink alcoholic beverages and eat a balanced diet will probably consume too many calories. If they drink but cut down on eating, they may not develop a weight problem, but they will probably develop nutritional deficiencies that can result in severe illness. Alcohol is also a central nervous system depressant, so it causes a decrease in one's metabolism.

In addition to the normal dangers of alcohol in creating alcoholism and destroying brain cells, there are other considerations in drinking. Beer or ale, because of their carbonation, have the effect of neutralizing stomach acid.

A FEW COMMON DRINKS AND THEIR CALORIC DAMAGE

BEVERAGE	SERVING SIZE	CALORIES	CARBS	FAT	PROTEIN	ALCOHOL
Bailey's Irish Cream, original	42 mL	137	11 g	5 g	1 g	6 g
Beer, regulary, industry average	341 mL	146	12 g	0 g	0 g	13 g
Beer, light, industry average	341 mL	99	5 g	0 g	0 g	11 g
Champagne	112 mL	84	2 g	0 g	0 g	11 g
Egg nog	222 mL	262	32 g	3 g	5 g	14 g
Martini, traditional	67 mL	124	1 g	0 g	0 g	18 g
Vodka, gin, rum, whisky	42 mL	97	0 g	0 g	0 g	14 g
Riesling	148 mL	118	6 g	0 g	0 g	14 g
Pino Grigio	148 mL	122	3 g	0 g	0 g	16 g
Merlot	148 mL	122	4 g	0 g	0 g	16 g
Red table wine, average	148 mL	125	4 g	0 g	0 g	16 g

SOURCE: MANUFACTURER'S WEBSITES, RETHINKINGDRINKING.NIAAA.NIH.GOV, USDA NUTRIENT DATABASE

JONATHON RIVAIT / NATIONAL POST

This might increase the acids secreted by the stomach, which could cause ulcers. Gin contains juniper berries and other substances that are stomach and intestinal irritants.

Studies have indicated that moderate alcohol consumption (less than 3 drinks a day) may increase the HDL type of blood cholesterol. There seems to be also a protective factor from a substance called resveratrol that is found in the seeds and skins of grapes. For that reason red wine would have even more protective qualities than other alcoholic drinks. Of course resveratrol can also be found in grape juice and in grapes, as well as in supplements, so there is no need to drink the wine to get the benefits. Before taking up drinking in order to reduce heart attack risk, one should consider that alcohol consumption is related to increased blood pressure and the added calories consumed may increase one's weight. Both of these are negatives in terms of heart disease.

Since Americans drink more beer than milk, 34 gallons a year per person for beer compared to 26 gallons per year per person for milk, health conscious people might consider drinking the best beverage, non-fat milk, rather than the more harmful alcohol.

FOOD ADDITIVES

Sugar is a negative for most people. In fact it is probably the most harmful additive to the foods that we in the United States eat. We average about 125 pounds of sugar per person per year. This gives us a lot of excess calories that, if we don't use for energy, we will store as fat. As discussed previously, if we exceed our desired weight and become obese, this will lead to increased health risks. While a few years ago sugar was suspected of creating hyperactivity in some children, it is now found not to be true according to the National Institute of Mental Health. (5)

Salt can be a dangerous additive to foods because people react differently to salt. Yet most people do not consider adding salt to their food a health risk. But when you look at populations as a whole, it seems obvious that the higher the salt intake, the greater the frequency of high blood pressure.

Since many manufacturers add salt to enhance the taste, sodium is often high. While the desired intake is between one and two grams (1,000 and 2,000 milligrams), the average intake in America is five grams (6) The potential negative effect of a high sodium intake can be combated by ingesting a high level of potassium. However, the desired recommended daily allowance for potassium, 2.5 grams, is not met by the average American, who consumes only 0.8 to 1.5 grams daily (Briggs, et al., p. 248). Most of our foods follow this same pattern -- too high in sodium and too low in potassium.

Preservatives added to foods give a longer storage life and prevent disease causing germs from multiplying. Most are harmless. Some give protection against intestinal cancers. And some, such as the nitrates in hot dogs, are cancer producing. However the disease of botulism, which they are preventing, is far more of a danger for disease than is the infinitesimal amount in the wiener.

Vitamins and minerals have been added to food for years. In 1917 Denmark began adding vitamin A to margarine because many children who did bot eat butter had developed serious eye problems. In 1973, the Food and Drug Administration suggested that more iron be added to enrich flour after they found that iron is often low in our diets. Vitamins A and D are often added to skim milk to make it non-fat milk--milk that has all of the nutrients of whole milk but without the fat. Vitamins A and D are fat soluble and stayed in the fat when the fat was removed to make the skim milk.

Vitamins oftentimes need to be added because they have been removed through processing. For example, white bread is often enriched with vitamins B1, B2 and B3. But this does not replace all of the B-complex vitamins that were removed when the food was processed. Pantothenic acid and folic acid, both B vitamins, are not present in the enriched foods but would be present in the natural foods such as whole grain bread. So, you should be aware that white bread is not the nutritional equivalent of whole grain bread. To be specific, it is lower in vitamin E, some of the B vitamins, and some of the trace minerals such as zinc and chromium than whole grain bread. However, whole grain bread contains phytic acid, which prevents the body from using iron, calcium and other minerals. So, there are positives and negatives to additives, processing, and other procedures used in modern food manufacturing

VEGETARIANISM

Vegetarianism is adhered to by people for two major reasons. Some have a reverence for life that precludes their eating of other animals. This is a belief prevalent in Hinduism. Since these vegetarians generally drink milk and may eat eggs, their diet may be nutritionally sound.

The second group of people are vegetarians for health reasons. They may believe that meat causes cancer or that there are harmful substances in meat or animal products including milk and eggs. Those vegetarians who do not consume any animal products or by-products are known as vegans. Their diets are often lacking in essential nutrients such as high quality protein, vitamin B12, vitamin D, calcium, and iron.

It has been found recently that many vegans are developing nutritional deficiency diseases such as rickets, pellagra, and scurvy. Medical records show irreversible physical and mental defects showing up in some children of such vegetarian parents.

Vegetarian diets that include milk or eggs can give proper nutrition if those animal proteins are taken in sufficient quantity. Cereal grains, beans, and nuts can also help to make up the essential amino acid deficiencies. Generally, a vegan needs 50 percent more total protein than others. This is still not insurance that all of the essential amino acids will be consumed because the amino acids are found in far better proportions in meat and dairy products than they are in fruits and vegetables.

When vegetarians are careful about their dietary intakes, they may prove to be healthier than non-vegetarians. One study compared healthy vegetarians to non-vegetarians and found that healthy vegetarians had lower blood sugar and cholesterol levels than did their closely-matched non-vegetarian counterparts (7)

SAVING ON THE FOOD DOLLAR

The consumer who wants to save money can save by being an intelligent shopper, an effective storer of food, and an imaginative cook who can minimize waste -- it is quite possible you will find that there are more economical, nutritious, and tasty ways of eating. But saving money will require some rethinking in your cooking and shopping requirements.

An expensive steak is not the best source of protein. Milk, an excellent source of high quality protein, and other protein-rich foods, can be combined to make a nutritious meal. Beans, rice, wheat, and corn are good protein-giving foods, but they must be combined with milk, eggs, or other animal products for maximum benefits.

Find cheaper sources of the same foods. Grass-fed beef is less expensive than grain-fed beef. By marinating the less-expensive cuts of meat and slicing them thin, a tasty dish can be served at a lesser price. Cheaper cuts of meat, such as beef or pork liver instead of calf liver, or round steak instead of top sirloin, can be acceptable substitutes if prepared correctly.

"Day old" bakery goods are just as nutritious as the freshly baked goods and may cost half as much. They can also be frozen and used later. Some of the bakeries that make non-fat desserts, such as cookies and cakes, also have such "day old" outlets.

Comparison shopping will probably show that there are "best buys" in nearly every grocery item. The identical quality may be less expensive in a different brand than that which you customarily buy. Clipping coupons can often save a great deal of money -- as long as you are buying items you really want.

Frozen orange juice and instant coffee are often less expensive than fresh oranges or ground coffee. On the other hand, prepared dishes, such as frozen spinach soufflés, are more expensive than making them from scratch.

Eggs, whether they are Grade A or Grade B, are equally nutritious. The difference is in the shape of their yolks. Egg whites have a very high quality of protein and should not be eliminated from most diets. However, if the eggs are soiled or cracked, they could be subject to food poisoning.

Another money-saving consideration is to buy fruit and vegetables in season when they are cheaper. In out-of-season times, canned or frozen items can be cheaper than fresh products. Take the time to compare prices before you make your purchasing decisions. To get the best value for your food, shop at stores that are neat and clean. There is a better chance that this is a better managed store and that the food is kept under proper conditions.

You can also save money by growing your own food. There are currently about 35,000,000 vegetable gardens under cultivation, 2 1/2 million more than a few years ago. Once you have harvested your food, you may find that canning it is the best way to preserve it. If you take proper precautions in canning, it can be an extremely effective way of preserving food.

If you're going to can your own foods, it's best to grow them at home. Your next best alternative in terms of cost is to buy them at a farm or roadside stand, while the most expensive is usually the supermarket. Make sure you know what you're doing when you're canning, because if it's done wrong, the food can either be ruined or botulism can occur.

If you decide to freeze your home-grown food, a Cornell University study has found that it costs as much as 19 cents a pound more than store-bought food. So freezing becomes a luxury. If you prefer to freeze food, choose a freezer that is not frost-free and restock it regularly. Frequent turnover cuts the costs. Invest in reusable containers. It will save money in the long run.

The average household wastes hundred dollars worth of food each year, according to researchers at the University of Arizona in Tucson. After several years of examining samples from household garbage collections, they discovered large amounts of food that could have been served as leftovers but had been thrown into the trash. The study didn't count food that was fed into the garbage disposals, dumped in compost piles, or fed to pets.

Imaginative cooking can be developed by consulting cookbooks specializing in the development of economical and tasty dishes. Leftovers from wilted lettuce to turkey bones can be used to make a nutritious stock for soups, stews, and casseroles. Microwave cooking is the least expensive way to cook. Crock pot cooking is next and oven use is the most expensive method of heating foods. While all cooking creates some free oxygen radicals, microwaving creates the least. The microwave is also useful for defrosting food.

Always use either the microwave oven or the refrigerator to defrost food. Putting frozen food on the counter invites the development of diseases.

When using your oven for cooking most foods, if you use heat-proof glass utensils, you can lower the oven setting by 25 degrees below that which is recommended for the cooking temperatures. This saves energy. If you are using your oven, cooking several dishes at the same time also lowers heating bills. Another hint -- don't peek at the food being cooked. Every time you open the oven door, as much as 20 percent of the heat can be lost.

If you find the cooking time for a food is over one hour, there's no need to preheat the oven even if the recipe calls for it. You may also find that foods that require a long cooking period can be cooked more efficiently in the oven than on the stove top because there is less heat loss in the oven. You'll also find that cooking foods such as meatloaf in muffin tins can reduce the cooking time by as much as 50 percent below that needed if it is cooked in a loaf.

Shopping for low fat foods requires a sharp eye. If you are looking for a low fat food, look at the total grams of fat, multiply by 9, then divide that by the total number of calories in the food. (For example, if there were 3 grams of fat times 9 calories in a gram of fat, this equals 27 total calories from fat. If the food had a total of 270 calories in it, then the percentage of fat calories is 10%.) If the food has one of the new food labels on it, all you need to do is divide the number of fat calories by the total number of calories for the food. This is how you calculate the approximate percentage of fat calories per serving. You want to keep your total percentage of fat below 30% everyday to decrease your risk of developing heart disease. 10 to 20% fat is better than the suggested maximum of 30%.

Many foods, particularly low fat liquids such as salad dressings without oil, have replaced the thickness of the oil with some gums. Guar, locust bean, and xanthine gums are soluble fibers so they help to remove cholesterol from the intestines. So, you get a double advantage --no fat in the dressing and some cholesterol removed from the intestines by the soluble fibers.

Evaluating your food. How you evaluate a food depends on your particular health concerns. If you are concerned with developing any type of cancer, you would want to reduce all fats. If you are concerned with decreasing your risk of heart disease, you would want to focus your attention on reducing saturated fats. If the fats come from animals, palm kernel oil, or coconut oil, they are saturated fats. Also, be on the lookout for hydrogenated fats (trans fatty acids) as this is a process that takes unsaturated fats and chemically saturates them. Trans-fats are illegal now in many areas of the world/If you are concerned with diabetes, you would want to check either the sugar content or the fats, depending on which caused you the problem. If you are worried about high blood pressure, you would want to check the sodium content.

The ingredients in the food must be listed according to their content in the product. The higher on the list of ingredients, the more of that item is present in the food. So, if the product lists wheat flour first, there is no problem. However, if it lists eggs or hydrogenated oils second, the food may be too high in fat. If you are on the lookout for sodium, remember to look for where salt is listed.

FOOD-RELATED DISEASES

There are many food-related diseases. Heart attacks and high blood pressure are sometimes triggered by an excess of salt or alcohol. Too much saturated fat or cholesterol in the diet can also increase one's risk of heart disease.

Obesity is a causative factor in diabetes, heart attack, and high blood pressure. This can be caused from too many calories in one's diet (usually from a high fat/high sugar diet), too little exercise, or a combination of both.

Cancers may also be caused to a degree by food. It seems that there is a great deal of evidence to indicate that cancers are primarily environmental and since the food we eat is part of our environment, it is highly probable that there may be cancers associated with food. All fats have been implicated as a higher risk for many cancers.

It has also been hypothesized that the high protein diet of most people in the United States is increasing their cancer rate. The reason would be that protein digestion produces an ammonia that can destroy cells. The incidence of cell turnover increases the chances of cells becoming cancerous. The ammonia also increases the risk of viral infection, and viruses are strongly suspected of being causative agents in some cancer production. This is merely a theory, but it can be taken into consideration.

Cancer of the large bowel is apparently linked to the high amount of refined food and the low amount of roughage in the average American's diet. Dr. Ernest Wynder, speaking to the American Cancer Society, estimated that half of the cancer deaths in women and 30 percent in men are related to nutrition.

Food-borne diseases affect 80 million Americans each year. Bacteria can breed easily in milk, eggs, and meat. Never mix old milk with new milk, because the developing bacteria in old milk can contaminate the new milk. Raw meat can also be a danger. It can carry live tape worms and trichinosis as well as salmonellosis.

, a common problem, is caused by bacteria found in meat, fish, poultry, and dairy products. It is estimated that two million people a year suffer from salmonella poisoning. Salmonella grows best in low-acid, moist food between the temperatures of 50° and 115°. Cooking at 160° destroys it. Symptoms of salmonella may include diarrhea, abdominal cramps, headache, chills, fever, and vomiting. The symptoms usually show up within 12 to 24 hours after ingesting the contaminated food, but symptoms may appear as soon as 6 hours or as long as 48 hours after food ingestion.

After preparing raw foods that might contain salmonella germs (including eggs, poultry, and meat), the cutting board should be thoroughly washed to kill any germs that might remain on the board. Cooked food should never be placed on an unwashed board that had been used for prior food preparation because salmonella germs might still be on it.

Some food poisoning is caused by the staphylococcus germs that live on people's skin and in their noses and throats. These can be transferred to the food by the people who are preparing it. This germ creates a toxin that inflames the stomach and intestines of the people who eat the tainted food. Symptoms of food poisoning caused by staphylococcus germs are similar to salmonellosis.

According to the Department of Agriculture, eggs, meat, fish, egg salad sandwiches, fried chicken, coleslaw, potato salad, or cream pies should not be "brown-bagged" to work or school, since they need constant refrigeration. If left unrefrigerated for only two to three hours, they can become a breeding ground for many disease-causing bacteria.

Several diseases can develop from eating raw mollusks (clams, oysters, mussels). They can be very dangerous--even when they are certified safe. These shellfish often live in water where they can pick up the coliform bacteria from human sewage. Each of these mollusks filters about 20 gallons of water a day through its system. If it lives in water that has live sewage in it, as do most coastal waters, they can harbor high amounts of these harmful bacteria. Even some cooked shell fish, such as steamed clams, can harbor the bacteria after being steamed.

Botulism is one of the most severe forms of food poisoning. The botulism bacteria grow only in surroundings in which there is no air and low acidity. The spores that produce botulism toxin can often be fatal. Although boiling kills most other living organisms, botulism bacteria are extremely resistant to heat. Botulism spores can be destroyed only when containers of low-acid foods are sterilized under pressure at temperatures high above the boiling point.

Botulism rarely occurs in commercially-canned foods. About 94 percent of the botulism cases previously seen were from home-canned foods. Since home canning has become more popular as the prices of various foods have gone up, doctors have observed an increase in the amount of botulism.

To minimize the dangers of botulism, food should be cooked in a pressure canner that reaches 240°F at 10 pounds pressure. Be particularly careful when canning meat, poultry, fish, and vegetables (except tomatoes or pickled vegetables). If you eat home-canned foods such as these, it is advised that you boil them for about 20 minutes after opening the jars. This should destroy any toxin present. Although it will ruin the texture of the vegetables, the food will not be poisonous.

Symptoms of botulism include double vision, difficulty in swallowing, dry mouth, constipation, and sometimes vomiting. They usually occur within 12 to 36 hours after ingesting the food and occasionally several days after eating the contaminated food. The death rate is high -- between 25 and 35 percent of those who contract it die.

Dental disease, primarily cavities, can be speeded up by two types of food -- food that forms plaque (the mucous-like covering over the teeth) and foods that contain high amounts of sugar. The plaque-forming foods give the bacteria on the teeth more area on which to grow. When bacteria consume the sugar, acid is formed that eats through the teeth.

Plaque-forming foods include oatmeal, pancakes, cakes, cookies, pies, ice cream, mayonnaise, candy, hot chocolate, milk shakes and canned fruit. Some foods can help reduce plaque. Foods that are high in fiber, such as fresh fruits and vegetables, can help to scrape plaque from the teeth.

HEALTH FOOD CLAIMS

Some health food stores push sea-salt as being a special kind of food additive that is better because it doesn't contain the iodine that the store-bought salt contains. This, of course, allows for the increased cost of this type of salt. Yet the iodine was added to the salt to prevent goiter, a thyroid gland enlarged because of the lack of iodine. So here again we see excess money spent for a lesser product.

Poisons added to foods are another area in which the health food people make claims. Poison is a relative term because the severity of one's reaction depends upon the amount ingested. For instance, arsenic in very small amounts may be medically beneficial, but in large amounts it is deadly. Also, aspirin in small amounts is often good, but an overdose would be fatal. In addition, strychnine is a severe poison, but in small amounts it can help people retain their memory. For any potential poison, two questions must be asked: what is the toxic level and is it cumulative in the body? Cumulative doses may develop tolerance, i.e., arsenic or heroin.

Health food sources suggest that chemical additives to foods are harmful. Preservatives, anti-oxidants, pesticides, and such are "bad." In actuality, this may not be true. For example, anti-oxidants help to cut down the presence of peroxide. It is known that some peroxides, such as rancid fats, are carcinogenic. We know that there is a very high frequency of stomach cancer in countries that do a lot of frying, reusing the same fat all the time. It has been hypothesized that a technological advance may be protecting us from cancer by adding the anti-oxidants. And as has been previously mentioned, the anti-oxidants reduce the dangerous free oxygen radicals.

Preservatives may decrease the amount of mold in certain foods. For example, aflatoxin is one of the most potent and dangerous carcinogens we know. It is produced by a common mold that grows in peanuts, corn, milk, bread, and many other foods. We protect ourselves against these toxins in part with mold inhibitors, a form of preservative. The large companies that make peanut butter use highly sophisticated machines to crack the outer and inner shells of the peanuts and then subject them to close scrutiny by photoelectric cells. Any discoloration of the peanuts activates an air jet that shoots the peanut off of the moving belt. We therefore eat peanut butter that is as free of mold as possible. But in Africa, where people eat all the peanuts, including those we know to be bad, there is a high rate of liver cancer. In this country, liver cancer (cancer that originates in the liver) is relatively rare.

The idea that every natural food is good may be questioned. There are toxins in mushrooms and bacteria in most natural foods. These naturally-occurring poisons are probably not harmful, but then neither are most, if not all, of the additives in "non-natural" foods. It is usually the dosage rather than the substance that is harmful in foods.

Pesticides, such as DDT, are other poisons considered bad by those who produce organic foods. However, pesticides are beneficial to farmers to enable them to produce a large crop without risking infestation. This allows more food to be produced and marketed to a hungry society. Also, a recent study of some New York health food stores revealed trace amounts of DDT found in their organic foods.

Organic foods have become more popular in the last several years, as people have become more concerned about their nutrition. There may be certain advantages to organic foods: they are often specially selected; they may have more eye appeal; and they have had limited or no insecticides used in their growing. But there are disadvantages also in that they cost more -- usually considerably more, and there are possible parasitic infections because of the lack of insecticides used.

Organically grown foods are claimed to be especially nutritious. One of the major claims of health food store owners is that they sell only organically-grown foods and that these foods are more nutritious than foods from grocery stores. Some doubt has been cast on these claims. For example, an organic carrot weighing 6 ounces will have the same number of nutrients as a non-organically grown carrot. It doesn't matter whether the nutrients were put into the ground by an animal fertilizer (organic foods) or a commercially made fertilizer.(8) There have also been newspaper articles challenging the claim that all the organically grown foods sold are actually organically grown because, according to their statistics, there appears to be more of such foods sold than grown.

Like in so many claims on both sides of the organic versus commercially grown products debate, there are questions relative to the truth of the arguments. For example, the conservative funded Center for Global Food Issues takes the side of commercial growing, while liberal groups, like the Union of Concerned Scientists criticize their evidence. The commercial interests charge that organic farming takes twice the land that commercial farming takes, especially for organic animals that have some freedom of movement. The extra land could be used for forests which would be better for the environment. A Danish study found that organic farming requires 25% more land than normal commercial farming. The liberal side counters that the food is healthier.

In looking at pluses and minuses of organic food versus what is called natural food, we find that organic food growers must agree to certain requirements in order to call their food "organic". Organic fruits and vegetables certainly cost more and do not seem to be any more nutritious than natural food. Some think they taste better, but taste may be dependent on freshness. Natural foods will have more pesticides than organic food but both will be in the safe category. Organic meats could be a different story. Grass fed beef has less fat than the grain fed beef. It isn't as juicy because it doesn't have as much fat. But it would be healthier to consume. When commercial farms use hormones and antibiotics to make the cattle bigger and more disease-free, it is conceivable that these hormones and antibiotics could harm the consumer. This isn't proven however.

Looking at organic versus commercial food from an environmental point of view we can see that organic farming uses more land to produce the same amount of food. This land might to be used to grow more food for starving people or to grow more trees to combat global warming. On the other hand organic farmers don't use pesticides so the earth is not polluted by absorbing them. Also organic farmers are more likely to rotate crops which might be environmentally advantageous.

Raw foods are also claimed to be better than cooked foods because the enzymes in the foods are not destroyed. This is false. The enzymes in uncooked food are destroyed by the body during digestion and are not absorbed into the body. Any value of raw foods would be in their increased water-soluble vitamin content and the structure of their fiber content.

Raw milk and pasteurized milk have the same nutrients, but raw milk contains certain enzymes that would otherwise be destroyed by pasteurization. There is a question as to whether these enzymes actually assist in effective nutrition. Raw milk may also contain many disease-causing organisms, including those for tuberculosis, undulant fever, and brucellosis. Certified dairies that produce raw milk are closely watched. Their cows are allowed a far lower bacterial count than is allowed to other commercial dairies. But the pasteurization of commercial milk brings its bacterial count to far below that of the certified raw milk product.

Raw eggs were consumed by the movie character "Rocky" in order to make him stronger. His nutritional knowledge did not compare to his boxing skill because those raw eggs were harder to digest than cooked eggs, and raw eggs often contain salmonellosis germs. Some food faddists say that the uncooked lecithin in raw eggs somehow neutralizes the cholesterol in the eggs, but this is not true.

Lecithin is taken by many people because it is extolled by the health food people. They believe it lowers blood cholesterol levels. This belief stems from experiments done over 30 years ago in which it was found that injected lecithin lowered blood cholesterol in some animals. Subsequent studies have shown that lecithin that is eaten has no such effect. The lecithin consumed by mouth is broken down into its component parts during the digestive process. There is no evidence that lecithin alone or lecithin combined with kelp or vinegar will do anything to make the blood vessels less clogged with fats.

Yogurt is a milk product that has been popularized in this country by the health food stores and is now sold in nearly every market. It is made from milk that has been predigested by a culture of bacteria. The major bacteria in yogurt are streptococcus thermophilus, lactobacillus acidophilus, and lactobacillus bulgaricus. When they are put together in milk at a temperature of about 110 degrees, they begin to break down the casein protein of the milk and also the lactose, which is a milk sugar. This lactose is then converted into lactic acid and acetaldehyde which is what gives the yogurt its distinctive flavor. The bacteria in the yogurt passes right through the body, so one would have to eat a cup of yogurt several times a day in order to keep a passable number of these living organisms in the intestines.

Yogurt has the advantage of being a digestible milk product for the many people who can't drink milk due to being lactose intolerant. However, for most people yogurt can be a poor buy for the amount of nutritional value received. If you are really fond of yogurt, it would be a wise investment to purchase a yogurt maker. (They cost between $15 and $25.) Not only will the resulting yogurt cost less (whatever the cost of the milk used) but there are possibilities for more personally satisfying flavors.

Honey is another food that is often suggested to be better than sugar because it has come from a natural source -- the bee. Honey is only sugar, and, as such, the body reacts to it in the same way that it reacts to refined sugar. Honey does bring with it other nutrients, but their health contributions are insignificant. In order to get one milligram of iron from honey, it would take five tablespoons of honey or 310 calories!

There is no real raw sugar in this country. Sugars sold in health food stores are just partially refined sugars. The darker the sugar, the less it has been refined. Brown sugar is not significantly better than white sugar. The molasses added to the sugar to make it brown adds few nutrients, and these are in very small quantities.

Fish oil pills may prove effective in reducing one's risk of developing heart and lung diseases. While it is generally recommended to eat the fish, thereby getting all of the high quality protein and minerals, ingesting pure fish oil may also be a positive health measure for some people. The omega 3 polyunsaturated oils have been shown to relax the arteries, making them larger (vasodilation). This increases the amount of oxygen available to the cells. Fish oils also slow the clotting time of the blood. And they reduce inflammation, possibly reducing the risk of atherosclerosis (9) They may also help people with lung problems, such as asthma, because they relax the muscles and open the airways. Of course, it is always wise to remember that oil, even fish oil, is fat and brings with it all of those extra calories.

The U.S. National Library of Medicine (10) has stated that fish oils, in pill form, can be valuable sources of omega-3 fatty acids. In salmon, herring, trout, sardines, tuna and mackerel—they are particularly abundant. It is recommended to eat fish at least three times a week. If you were to rely on fish oil pills, you would want to make sure that you got at least three or four grams a week. Fish oil pills generally have a third to a half gram of omega-3s, so you need to check the label to see how many pills a week you would need. There are several types of omega-3 fatty acids. Two of the most important omega-3 fatty acids contained in fish oil are eicosapentaenoic acid (EPA) and docosahexaenoic acid (DHA).

Research indicates that omega-3 fatty acids are effective for lowering blood triglycerides, which are associated with heart disease and untreated diabetes. The omega-3s are likely beneficial in preventing heart disease and heart attacks. It is possible that they may lower blood pressure, reduce the pain of rheumatoid arthritis and menstrual pain. They may also be useful in improving the thinking skills of children with ADHD. They may also be useful in preventing stroke, osteoporosis (weakened bones), hardening of the arteries and kidney problems. There may also be mental advantages. Omega-3s have been noted to reduce depression, and psychosis, including bipolar disorders.

With all its potential benefits, many claims have been made for it that have not been verified, such as: preventing headaches, preventing liver disease, treatment for ulcers and other physical problems.

While fish oil pills are safe at doses of less than three grams per day, more than that could cause problems such as: bleeding, due to the reduced clotting ability of the blood; high doses might reduce the effectiveness of the immune system which could reduce the body's effectiveness in fighting infections; it might even increase the levels of bad cholesterol (LDL) in some people; fish oil from the larger fish can be contaminated with mercury or other chemicals but fish oil pills should not have this problem. There are some other possible problems, so you should check with your doctor to see if fish oil pills would be a plus or minus for your health.

EATING AND OVEREATING

Obviously people eat to nourish their bodies. But in America many people eat as a means of reducing stress. We may not be satiated in our work, at school, or in our relationships but we can be satiated with food. Filling our stomachs can make us feel that in at least one part of our lives we are totally satisfied. When eating to relieve stress we will probably take in more calories than we need for living, but worse, stress eating is often done with junk foods. Chocolate, ice cream, French fries, or pastries are doubly satisfying because they taste so good while they fill us up.

Why do you eat? At least part of your answer lies in the feeding center of your brain. When you begin to eat, the sugar content of the blood goes up, and the hypothalamus turns off. It also secretes a hormone that signals to your brain when you have had enough. This part of your hunger comes from your biological clock. In your daily routine, you expect to eat at certain times of the day. If you go through the lunch hour without eating, you will be very hungry at the time, but as time passes, you will generally become less hungry. The hunger pangs that come from stomach contractions are learned and almost any habit that is learned can be unlearned if you go about it in the right way

If you were to go without eating, the experience of hunger will rise to a maximum in three to five days as the brain and stomach muscles continue to learn that the food supply has stopped. The stomach contractions will slow down and eventually cease almost entirely. Your body can be trained not to be hungry. The first three days of starvation or the first three days of a diet (when you reduce your caloric intake to lose weight) are the worst. It isn't that your stomach shrinks, it is that you learn to not be hungry and your hypothalamus learns to adjust to the new, lower blood sugar levels.

Gaining weight is a desire for some people. When one focuses on weight gain, he or she is focused on increasing his or her lean body weight. This means that one wants to increase one's weight by increasing muscle mass, not fat. To gain weight in muscle, the best method is to do resistance-type exercise, such as weight training. Second, you must ensure that you are eating enough protein in order to give your body the building blocks that it needs to make more muscle. It is not necessary to eat excessive protein, as this dietary practice brings with it its own set of health risks (11)

OBESITY AND OVERWEIGHT

There is no question that you have heard about the epidemic of overweight and obesity in the Western world. And you know it is being led by the United States. The most common measure today for evaluating overweight and obesity is the BMI—body mass index. It is the relationship between your height and your weight. There are several ways to calculate it depending on whether you use pounds and inches, kilograms and meters or, in England, stones and inches. Those with a BMI over 30 are considered to be obese.

There are some criticisms of the BMI. Heavily muscled people will often be categorized as obese. Older people will generally have lost muscle and added fat without much of a change in weight. There is also evidence of racial and ethnic variations from the mainly Caucasian based BMI. Still all excess weight may be a negative factor in longevity—excess fat is far worse than excess muscle.

However, the BMI is today's standard and using it we find that in the U.S. about one in three adults (33.8%) is obese and 12.6 million children and adolescents (17%) are obese. The increase is alarming. Here are the most recent ratings by state.

Studies in the US over the last few decades have shown an alarmingly increasing amount of overweight and obesity throughout the US. Similar patterns are being shown in Europe, but they are about 10 to 20 years slower than the US in developing these patterns of obesity.

Obesity Trends* Among U.S. Adults
BRFSS, 1990, 2000, 2010
(*BMI ≥30, or about 30 lbs. overweight for 5'4" person)

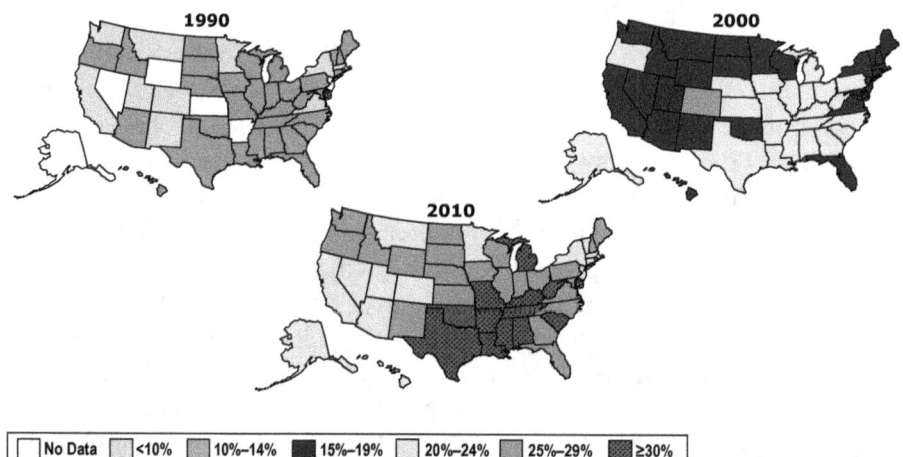

| No Data | <10% | 10%–14% | 15%–19% | 20%–24% | 25%–29% | ≥30% |

In the US, or countries using the Imperial standard, you would divide your weight in pounds, multiplied by 703, by your height, in inches squared. So your BMI would be:

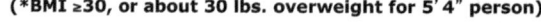

$$\frac{\text{weight in pounds} \times 703}{(\text{height in inches})^2}$$

If you live in a country that uses the metric system you would divide your body weight in kilograms by height in meters squared.

$$\frac{\text{your weight in kilograms}}{(\text{your height in meters})^2}$$

The simplest way to figure it is to go to a search engine on your computer and search for "BMI and calculate.' Or to make a less accurate but simple estimate, check the charts below.

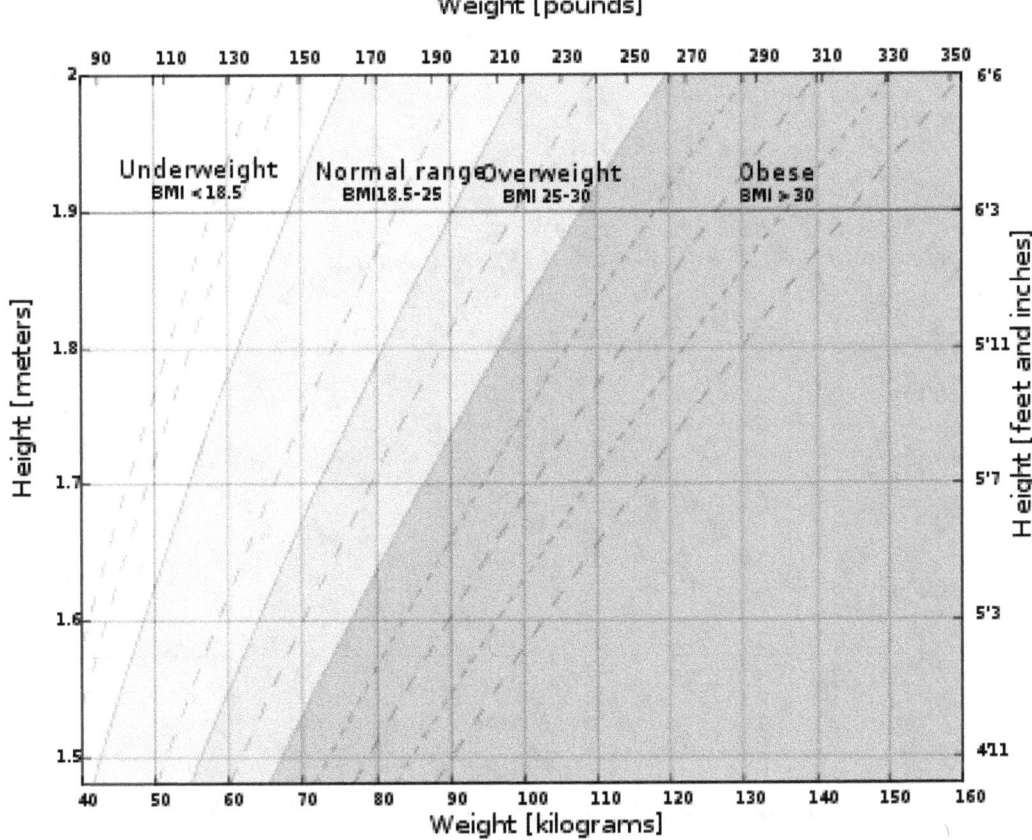

Being overweight can kill you! In 2010 a combination of 19 long-term studies, ranging from 5 to 28 years and involving over 1 ½ million primarily Caucasian adults, concluded that even being a bit overweight is risky. Healthy adults who were above the normal range for their BMIs were 13% more likely to die. The meta-analysis was done by the American Cancer Society. (12)

Being overweight increases one's chances of dying by 13%. Being obese increased one's chance of dying by 44, 88 and 250%, depending on how obese the person was. The people with the greatest chance of living were in the high end of the normal range, with BMIs of 22.5 to 24.9. The studies excluded people who smoked, or had heart disease or cancer and they did not measure physical fitness or nutritional status.

The National Center for Health Statistics now finds that 34% 0f Americans are obese, including 6% who are extremely obese, and 32.7% are overweight, The World Health Organization further divides BMI groups.

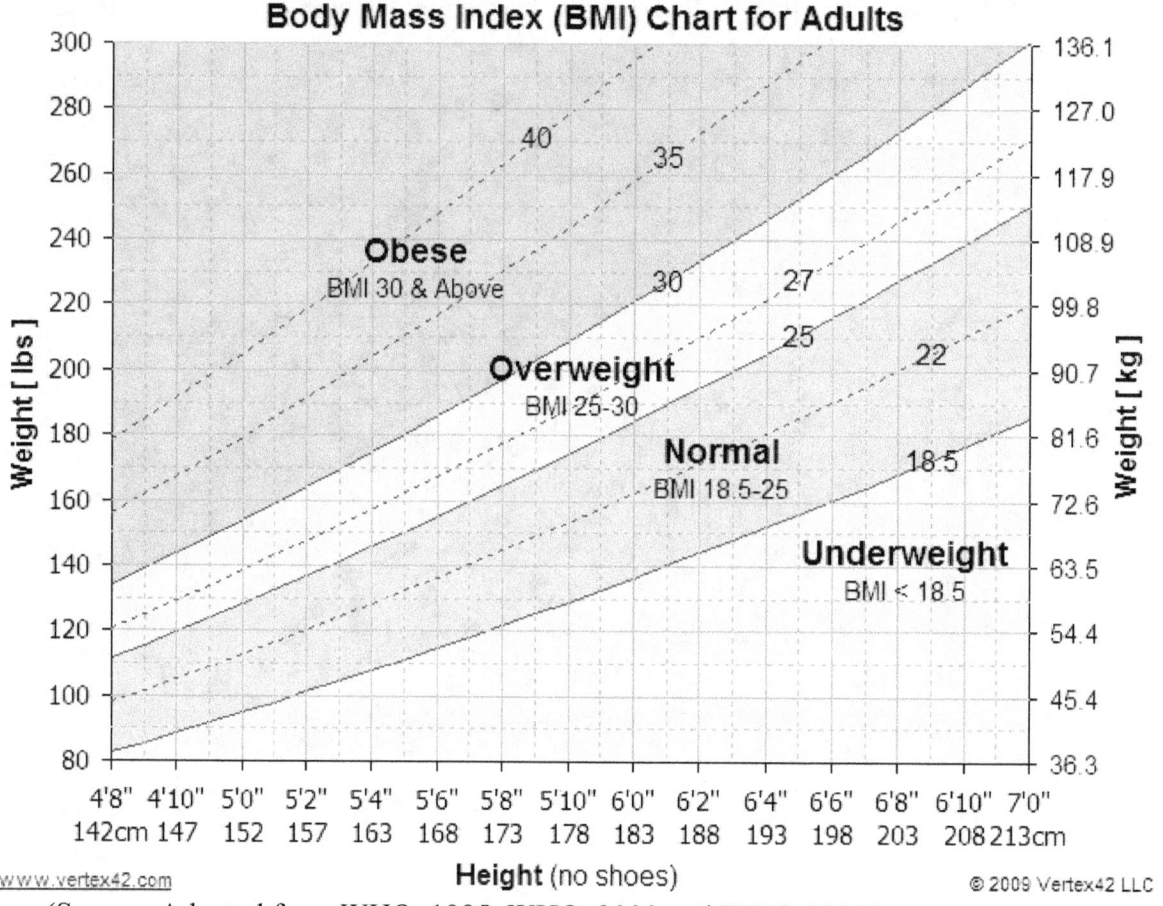

Body Mass Index (BMI) Chart for Adults

(Source: Adapted from WHO, 1995, WHO, 2000 and WHO 2004.)

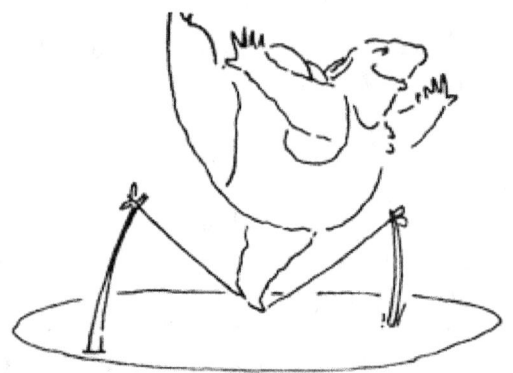

Dieting isn't for everyone. Some people function better when they are fat.
HILDE BRUCHE, PROFESSOR OF PSYCHIATRY

Of the people who are obese, one in 20 is so because of a genetic factor or a problem in physical malfunctioning, such as an underactive thyroid, a problem with the hypothalamus, or one of the other centers of the brain that deals with whether or not we feel full or hungry. There are medical procedures that can help these people. In cases where the metabolism is slowed, such as by an underactive thyroid gland, doctors can administer the proper hormone to increase metabolism back into what is considered a "normal" range.

Studies of twins raised in different households show a strong hereditary link to obesity. One cause of obesity has been recently found in a gene that signals the brain that the person has had enough to eat. If that gene is defective the person may eat much more than the body needs.

Another tendency toward being obese is thought to be caused by the number of fat cells in a person's body. This is known as the set point theory. It is thought that the more fat cells one has, the more one is driven to eat to maintain these fat cells. The number of fat cells one has is generally set after puberty—but can be increased by overeating. Fat cells can increase in size to a maximum size, then new fat cells can be developed from cells called fibroblasts. Once in place fat cells don't seem to be capable disappearing. They merely get larger or smaller. After this, it is the size of the fat cells that changes to accommodate fluctuations is one's weight. Fat cells in an obese person may be three times as large as those in a lean person. Dieting may make the fat cells reduce in size, but not in number. The thinner cells just sit around waiting to be fed.

For others, obesity can be caused by overeating to an extreme degree. However, according to the Harvard University Nutrition Department, most people who are overfat are overfat because they lack exercise, not because they overeat. Overeating coupled with a lack of exercise is a sure way of becoming obese.

Since it is the amount of fat that a person carries on his/her body that is a major culprit of disease, it is preferable to refer to being overfat as a health risk rather than being overweight. Many body builders may be overweight when compared to the height/weight charts commonly used to measure health risks by insurance companies, but they are not overfat.

OTHER MEASUREMENT FOR DETERMINING OVERFAT

Determining if you are overfat can be done in other ways than determining one's BMI. The most common method is to look at yourself in a mirror. If you look fat, you may be fat—unless you are an anorexic!. Another way is to pinch the fat you carry just below the skin. If you can pinch an inch, you are probably carrying too much fat.

Professionals often use skin calipers to measure the amount of fat people carry in seven designated spots on the body (i.e. front and back of the upper arm, upper chest, upper back, stomach, hip, and front of the thigh). The sum of these skinfolds will be used to determine an overall percentage of body fat for you. Because men carry their fat predominantly around the waist, while a woman's fat is distributed mostly in the thighs and buttock area, there are different sites of measurement for men and women. The most accurate way to measure one's percent of body fat is with underwater weighing. This method is only available in high level testing labs. Another method is bioelectrical impedance, which measures the amount of fat and lean body mass via an electrical current that is sent through the body. This method is greatly influenced by such things as caffeine and alcohol ingestion which can throw off the accuracy of the test results.

Once your body fat percentage is determined, you can then find out what a healthy weight would be for you. Men are usually considered healthy if their body fat is in the range of 10 to 15%, while women are healthy if they fall between 18 and 25% body fat. Men are considered overfat if their body fat is over 20%, while women are overfat if their body fat is over 30%. Women require more fat than do men due to the menstrual cycle. If a woman falls below 12% body fat, she may become amenorrheic (lose her regular menstrual cycle).

For many years the Metropolitan Life Insurance Company has published the results of an extensive evaluation by the Society of Actuaries. This study resulted in the production of a table of desired weights based on one's weight (dressed, 3 pounds of clothes for women, 5 pounds for men), height (with 1 inch heeled shoes) and body frame (estimated by the width of the elbow). The risk of dying was dependent only on one's weight, while we might assume that being overfat was the primary reason for being overweight, these charts only take into consideration one's total weight.

Click for tables. https://www.bcbst.com/MPManual/HW.htm

Another concern for your health risk is where you store your fat. Those who store their fat in the abdomen, thereby resembling an "apple" shape, are at a higher risk for developing heart disease than those who store their fat in the hips and thighs, thereby resembling a "pear" shape. So, if two men have the same percentage of body fat but different shapes, the one who is "apple" shaped is at a greater risk than the "pear", even though their percentage of body fat is the same. As you may have noticed, most men tend to be "apple" shaped, while most women tend to be "pear" shaped. Thus, most women are at a lower risk than most men, simply because of where they store their fat.

THE DANGERS OF BEING OVERFAT

Those who are overfat can develop many problems such as osteoarthritis (from excessive wearing of the joints due to the continual carrying of excess weight), Type 2 diabetes (from excessive blood sugar), high blood pressure, and hardening of the arteries—both of which are responsible for heart disease and stroke, some cancers and sleep apnea. It also contributes to gall bladder disease, fatty liver disease and complications during pregnancy. Being overfat will probably speed up our death. There is evidence to indicate that perhaps fat people live faster than thin people. Studies with rats have found that the fat rat babies lived faster. They reached sexual maturity faster, ran sooner, and even died earlier than normal-weight rats.

In addition to the physical health risks, our society has placed additional psychological reasons for not being obese. Unhappily dieting has become a way of life for many Americans. It seems that being overweight is often considered to be a character flaw. It is a sad commentary, but the realities are that being obese often reduces a person's self esteem and often dooms them to lower socio-economic classes and reduces their chances for greater education and higher paying jobs. It also reduces one's chance of marrying.

A recent study at George Washington University, summarizing other studies, calculated additional financial costs to being obese. It found an annual cost of $4,879 for women and $2,646 for men. It included the costs of being in a lower wage earning job, for women, the cost of sick days, increased medical expenses (about $1400 a year) and several other expenses.

SHOULD YOU LOSE WEIGHT?

Before you decide to lose weight, you first need to determine whether your are overweight due to being overfat. From a health point of view it is your proportion of fat and lean body mass that is most important.

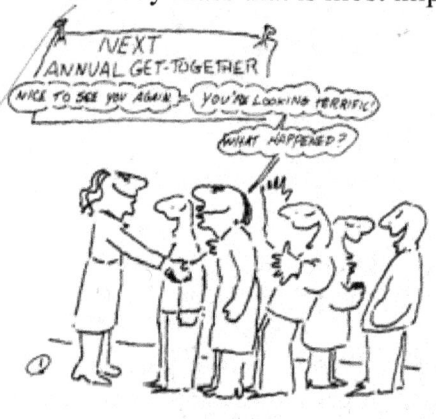

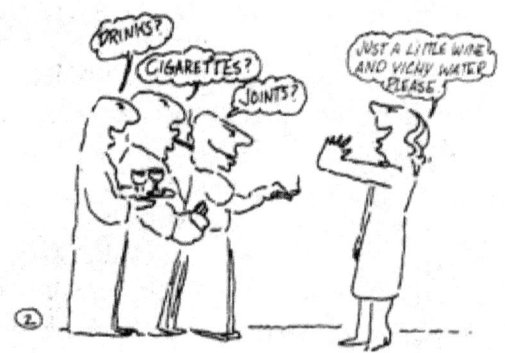

80

The wisest approach to losing weight would be to find out why you are overweight. If it is genetic, perhaps medical help is needed. If you eat because of stresses you should find another method to relieve the stresses, such as exercise or relaxation techniques or, if you must have something in your mouth, try gum or a low calorie food. If your problem is a lack of exercise, obviously you should start an effective exercise program. If it is that you consume too many calories, you will need to change your diet.

Determining what needs to be done is the first step toward successful dieting. The next decision is the value question --what is more important, my self centered desire to put food in my mouth now--at the present time, or the self centered value in which the future is more important. The reasons for the future value would be living longer, feeling better, and having a better body image. For most people it is the self centered, present time, value that directs a large part of their lives. That is why a dieter may indulge in a hot fudge sundae, a half dozen donuts, or a couple of beers, knowing that such behavior is counter to the long term goal of permanent weight loss. The seriousness of your commitment is primary.

Don't even start a weight loss program if you are not willing to make lifestyle changes for the rest of your life. The great majority of dieters refuse to make such a commitment. That is why 40% of women and 25% of men are on a diet at any one time and that the average American goes on 2.3 diets a year and why 95% of dieters have regained all of their lost weight within five years. The average diet is just not successful.

In all likelihood, adopting the habits of effective exercise and a low fat and low alcohol eating pattern, the pounds will drop off. Losing weight, just for the sake of being thinner, seldom works for very long. Consequently you will have to determine whether you honestly want a healthier lifestyle or you just want to look better for the summer. A pattern of continually gaining and losing is frustrating and probably not worth the effort. But a true lifestyle change of healthy eating and effective exercise will pay many mental, physical, and social dividends.

We must recognize that the fat we wear comes primarily from the fat we eat. Because of the efficiency of conversion to the sugar glucose, carbohydrates are used first for energy in the body. To convert carbohydrates to fat requires about 23% of the energy to be used to make the conversion. Protein, if not used to build tissues, will normally be converted into sugars and will be the second source of available energy. But fat which you have consumed uses only 3% of its food value to convert it to body fat. (14)

So 25 grams of carbohydrate, which will yield 100 calories (at 4 calories a gram) is reduced by 23% of the calories when used to convert them to body fat. But fats consumed in your food are different. 11 grams of fat (at 9 calories per gram) is 99 calories but it only takes 3% of those calories to convert it all to body fat. Consequently 96 calories of body fat can be deposited. So approximately 100 grams of carbohydrate, if not used for energy, will become 8.5 grams of body fat but a 100 grams of fat, if not used for energy, will become 10.75 grams of body fat.

Yo-yo dieters are those who lose then gain, then lose and gain, again and again. This type of dieting behavior will be at best discouraging, and at worst, harmful. Some researchers have found that if one's metabolism is continually decreased over time with repeated diets it will be reduced permanently. People who have been on starvation diets may find that their metabolism drops. This was especially true in Nazi prison camps where the imprisoned Jews, living on far below starvation levels of calories, were still able to survive because their metabolism levels dropped. This drop seemed to be relatively permanent after they left the concentration camps. So, if you start out with a low metabolism and engage in yo-yo dieting, you run the risk of lowering your metabolism even further.

When you diet, both fat and muscle are lost. When the weight is allowed to return to pre-diet levels, it is almost all in fat. Then the next diet begins. Again both muscle and fat are lost. With the next weight gain more fat is put on. So the person, after a series of such diets, is fatter than before even though the weight is the same. In addition to the increase in fat, there is a corresponding decrease in lean body tissue, leading to an overall decrease in metabolism (it is your lean tissue that uses energy all the time, not your fat cells). Yo-yo dieting is not an effective way to lose weight and keep it off, but it is not harmful to one's health. (16)

In order to make weight loss permanent, you must have a plan that will give you a lifelong change of habits. You will have to make certain that you have the proper amount of protein (about half of a gram of protein for every pound of body weight), your fat consumption should be low (preferably in the 10 to 20% range of fat calories as a percentage of total calories), and you should have an array of complex carbohydrates to give you the vitamins, minerals, and fiber that you need. You may want to add vitamin and mineral supplements to make certain that you have these nutrients at the optimal levels.

To aid in your pursuit of weight loss, you may decide to change your eating habits. It is a good idea to eat smaller, more frequent meals rather than infrequent, large meals. Every time you eat, you increase your metabolism because you put your digestive system to work. There is evidence that eating four or five small meals a day is better than eating two or three large ones. It also seems to reduce the cholesterol level of the blood.

Another approach to dieting is to eliminate some foods at some meals -- instead of having potatoes every night, have them every other night. Or you may decide to have open-faced sandwiches instead of sandwiches with two slices of bread. (Some people use lettuce leaves instead of bread to make a sandwich.) Switching from meat to poultry or fish and from regular ice cream to a "light" frozen dessert can save you calories while maintaining your nutritional status.

For permanent weight loss, you want to lose about one pound of fat per week, no more than two pounds of body weight. The best way to lose weight permanently is to combine an aerobic exercise program (to burn fat and increase your metabolism) with a diet that is close to the diet you will maintain once you have reached your goal weight.

Exercise must be a part of a healthy weight loss and weight maintenance program. It is wise to begin a weight training program because you will want to increase muscle size so that you gain muscle while you lose fat. Normally when people diet they lose both fat and muscle. You don't want that. Muscle is more metabolically active. A pound of muscle uses more calories per hour than does a pound of fat.

When you exercise you increase your metabolism, so you use more calories. Everyone knows that. What many don't know is that after exercising you burn more calories for the next hour or day—depending on the length and intensity of the exercise. Running a marathon will burn extra calories for nearly two days. Walking for fifteen minutes will use more calories for the next hour or two. A study in Japan showed that 30 minutes of exercise when done in three 10 minute bouts, separated by 10 minute rest periods used more calories than doing the same exercise at the same intensity for 30 minutes uninterrupted. (17)

While the recommended minimum weekly exercise program is 30 to 45 minutes three to five days a week (18) Anything is better than nothing. Even 15 minutes a day of walking has positive effects on reducing heart disease, but 45 minutes daily is better. If you are really intent on burning fat, an hour a day of uninterrupted exercise seems to be a good idea. That bit of information might be valuable for Sylvester Stallone or Arnold Schwarzenegger who must drop some fat for the next "super buff" movie role, but it may be a bit extreme for most of us. It would be wisest, however, to use shorter but more frequent bouts of exercise during the day. For college students, a brisk walk between classes would be better than a leisurely stroll. For an office worker, 15 minute walks at coffee break time and lunch would be wise. And for the housewife or house-husband spacing a brisk vacuuming session, a shopping trip and a walk to pick up the kids at school would make more sense than doing them all at about the same time then resting the remainder of the day. You might also think of parking the car two blocks from the school then walking. That's better for the kids too!

To lose one pound of fat per week, you must have a net deficit of 500 calories per day. This is because one pound of fat contains 3,500 calories. You may choose to achieve this solely by decreasing your food intake by 500 calories per day. However, if this is your approach, be warned: your metabolism will slowly decrease over time to accommodate for the decrease in food energy, thereby making it harder and harder for you to continue to lose fat.

You could also choose to increase your activity level to burn off 500 calories a day. Keep in mind that it takes a great deal of energy to achieve this goal, and it can be dangerous for you to embark on such a strenuous exercise program if you are currently not exercising. Therefore, it is best to combine both calorie reduction with exercise to achieve your goal. Aerobic exercise will keep your metabolism up as you lose the fat, and you won't have to restrict your calories to such an extreme because you will be burning off energy each time you exercise. Strength training will reduce the amount of muscle that might be lost in dieting and may actually increase the total amount of muscle tissue.

The number of calories you use depends on your weight and on the type of exercise you do. If you weigh 150 pounds, you would use about 60 calories just sitting and watching TV for an hour. So that hour of sitting will work off the calories in a chocolate chip cookie. If our days were 100 hours long, watching TV might be an effective method of losing weight. A problem is that most people munch while tube viewing so it is generally a double negative. One study showed that for children it was the eating while watching that put on the weight. Those who did not eat while watching TV did not generally have a weight problem.

On the other hand, if you are playing aggressive soccer or doing a high impact aerobic dance workout you might use 4 to 6 times as many calories as you would watching TV. With a chocolate chip cookie having 50 to 100 calories in it, you can get an idea of how much exercise you need to do to burn off one cookie. (At the end of the chapter a long list of activities, both recreational and vocational, is presented. This will give you an idea of the number of calories used in different activities.)

It is becoming more common to ride an exercise bike while watching TV at home. As the commercial gyms have found, watching TV while walking a treadmill or pedaling an exercise bike is more enjoyable for most of us.

Some people think that exercising will make them eat more. A quarter mile to a mile of jogging will have no measurable effect on the total intake of calories. In fact, by exercising just before a meal, you can dull your appetite and decrease your desire for more calories.

At any rate you must realize that permanent weight loss is a slow process -- remember how long it took you to put on those extra pounds!

Behavior modification is another approach to weight loss. This approach is advocated by the behaviorist school of psychology. Several things can be done in an attempt to modify one's behavior. First, the person has to become aware of how much food is being eaten. It takes about 20 minutes for the stomach to inform the brain, by signals from the hypothalamus, that it has had enough food. If a person eats slowly for the first 20 minutes of a meal, the time can be used to turn the brain off before a great deal of food is eaten. Secondly, a person may learn to savor the food differently by becoming conscious of the taste. Enjoy every bite, perhaps setting the fork down between bites. People can also learn to substitute food, such as a big salad and clear broth for sweets and fatty meats.

Before you can change your eating habits, you must be aware of exactly what you are doing. Behavior modification experts generally suggest that you keep a food diary for at least a week. The diary is to include of everything you eat and drink, the time you eat, what you were doing while eating, and the feelings you were experiencing at that time. You may find that you feel the urge to eat while you are studying, or when the television is on, or whenever you pass the refrigerator. Also, some require that you include who was near you at the time you ate.

After you have completed your food diary, look for patterns in your behavior. Do you like to eat in bed? Do you eat in your car, or while you are in the kitchen? If so, you may have to modify your behavior to eliminate these places. You might make a rule that you will eat only while sitting at the dining room table with the TV turned off. Or maybe your rule would be that you will snack only in the hall. The idea of this is to make you aware of the behavior patterns you have established -- so that you are conscious of when, where, and why you are eating – then to change those patterns.

People who carry excess weight tend to be more subject to external cues in their eating habits. When presented with a fear situation, overfat people ate about the same amount of food that they would normally eat, while those in the desirable weight range ate less food. When told it was past their dinner time, overly fat people would eat more than normal, while healthy weight people would not eat, or eat very little, unless they were hungry.

Another helpful hint may be to change your eating times. Instead of breakfast at 7, lunch at 12, and dinner at 6, you may try to fool your hypothalamus and stomach muscles. Let your stomach growl at 7, then eat something at 8. Then you might try having a small lunch at 11:30. Your stomach should be too embarrassed to growl at 12. You might sneak a snack at 5 and fool your hypothalamus again. Since we have been conditioned, like Pavlov's dogs, to eat at certain times, we often need to unlearn these habits.

For some people, it may help to tell the world about your weight loss plan to gain additional encouragement. Also, you may be less apt to quit if you have all those people to deal with later. For others, telling the world may not be a good idea. If you prefer to keep it to yourself, then do. You are not required to tell anyone of the changes you intend to make in yourself. Regardless of who you decide to tell, enjoy the compliments that come your way as you slowly attain your goal, and realize that you've earned them.

You might involve yourself with other people with similar weight loss goals. This is why Overeaters Anonymous and Weight Watchers are effective. You will be able to reward others, and they can reward you as your weight loss progresses.

You can use other psychological cues when dieting. You might put up a chart to list your daily food intake and exercise program. You may also want to chart your weight every week. Remember, only you can be responsible for your weight loss, and it is up to you to take control of it. It is a good idea to set up both short and long-term goals for yourself, and reward yourself every time you reach a goal. Keep in mind that a reward of a hot fudge sundae may not be the most effective reward!

Setting weight loss goals is generally a good idea. It is wise to set small weight loss goals, rather then saying, "I'm going to lose 70 pounds." Set a goal of three or five pounds. When this goal is attained, give yourself a reward. This way you'll get many senses of success while on your way to achieving your ultimate weight loss goal. Losing even one pound is a tough job, so don't let that go unnoticed. Many short-term goals accompanied by rewards help to keep up your motivation and stay on track.

A sensible weight loss diet requires maintaining good nutrition. It is important to remember that, even when eating to lose weight, you must give your body the nutrients that it needs. You must not compound your weight problem by inadequate nutrition while eating fewer calories, or your body will slip into starvation mode thereby lowering your metabolism in its attempt to store fat.

Usually reducing your intake of fat (which saves nine calories per gram), alcohol (which saves 7 calories per gram), and some carbohydrates—especially the sweets (which saves four calories per gram) will result in successful weight loss. Alcohol is a major stumbling block to dieters. Not only does it contribute 7 calories per gram, that's 170 calories for a bottle of beer, but because it is a depressant, it slows the body's metabolism. A person consuming 25% of his or her calories from alcohol reduces the body's ability to burn fat by 33%. (19)

Glycemic Indexes and Glycemic Loads for Common Foods

It is very easy to add calories. But, if you know where to look, you'll be able to avoid many calorie traps. For example, a potato is not a bad thing to eat if it is baked or boiled by itself (100 calories). If it's mashed with whole milk, a serving increases to 150 calories. When butter and cream are added, the total calories shoots up to 250 (the same as French fries). For that same 100 calorie potato, hash browns jump your calories up to 400 to 500 calories per serving because of the oil used in frying. So, try to avoid fried foods as this skyrockets your fat intake. For most foods, choose those that are baked or broiled to help save yourself from those sneaky calories. Reducing sweets, while it may not be palatable, is one of the most effective ways of limiting calories.

THE GLYCEMIC INDEX

In evaluating carbohydrates, those with a high glycemic index, the carbohydrates that quickly break down into glycogen (simple sugar) are not recommended. This is particularly true for those people who suffer from hypoglycemia—low blood sugar. For these people the glycemic index is important. While only about 5% of the general population has it, nearly 50% of diabetics may have problems with it. And since nearly 12% of the population has diabetes or pre-diabetic conditions, we can estimate that perhaps 10 or 11% of people may be bothered by hypoglycemia.

While a high glycemic index food will raise one's blood sugar level quickly, it is desirable to have a more constant blood sugar level, so foods that break down into energy more slowly, like proteins and complex carbohydrates, make much more sense from a health point of view.

What foods are high, and undesirable, for hypoglycemia? Low and behold!—ice cream, white bread and white rice are high. Non-fat milk and broccoli are low and whole grain bread is much lower than white bread. Here is a look at a few foods and their glycemic indices. (See a listing of the glycemic indices of more foods at the end of the chapter.)

Our old habits die hard, but often changes can be made. If you drink soft drinks, use the diet variety--even if it doesn't taste quite as good. Have your vegetable salad with a non-fat dressing. Take the skin off of the chicken and save all of those fat calories. Forget the butter on the bread. Use non-fat products whenever possible. Eat more fruits and vegetables. Broil your meats. In other words, think about what is best--not what is usual--for you.

SUMMARY OF DIET IDEAS

1. Plan an eating change in which you reduce your daily calories by 500 in order to lose a pound a week.

2. Achieve this reduction by reducing fats and alcohol and eating smaller portions of food or eliminating some foods from some meals.

3. Add aerobic exercise to your life--swimming, walking, jogging, cycling at a level sufficient to expend at least 500 calories a week. (See the fitness chapter.)

4. Consider spreading your calories into several meals rather than the traditional three meals a day.

THE BEST DIET FOR WEIGHT LOSS

A recent study from Denmark using 1200 adults from eight European countries in the "Diet, Obesity, and Genes (Diogenes) Project" (20) had the subjects divided into four diet categories: a low-protein and low-glycemic-index diet, a low-protein and high-glycemic-index diet, a high-protein and low-glycemic-index diet, a high-protein and high-glycemic-index diet, or a control diet. To promote weight loss and inhibit the regaining of weight the high protein-low glycemic index diet was best. The low protein-high glycemic index diet was worst.

Strange that the best weight loss diet is about the same as the best diet for health! High quality protein (egg whites, non-fat milk, fish and skinless poultry, whole grain products, and whole fruits and vegetables.

If you are seriously interested in intelligently analyzing your diet it is suggested that your buy a copy of the book Bowes & Church's Food Values of Portions Commonly Used. Amazon.com sells it new for $35 and used for $2. Older editions are fine. The Department of Agriculture has a publication that is nowhere near as complete, but it is free on the Internet. Search: Nutritive Value of Foods.

ADDITIONAL MATERIAL

GLOSSARY

*Prostaglandins are hormone-like substances produced in the body. Insulin and epinephrine are examples.

*Thromboxane a prostaglandin made from arachidonic acid an essential fatty acid.

*Actuaries. Insurance company employees who deal with probabilities of death, in juries, or accidents.

*Biological clock. Many organisms tend to develop habits as if they were controlled by a clock inside their biological beings. This "clock" seems to be guided by the longitude in which the organism lives. For example, people tend to wake up at their accustomed time, whether or not it is light outside. They tend to become hungry at their accustomed hours of eating even if there is no physiological reason for their hunger. Once the accustomed eating time is past, the stomach muscles may not exhibit hunger, even though o person has not eaten.

*Carcinogenic. Cancer producing.

*Goiter (goy-ter). An enlargement of the thyroid gland.

*Hypothalamus (hi-po-thal-a-mus). A part of the brain which stimulates many body functions.

*Ketones. Breakdown products of fats.

*Lactobacillus bulgaricus (lak-to-ba-sil-is bul-gar-i-kus)

*Nitrates. Some as above, but potentially more harmful than nitrites .

*Nitrites. Food preservatives, which may be cancer producing when combined with other substances.

*Obese (o-bes). Excessively fat, usually defined as 20% over ideal body weight.

*Parasitic (par-a-sit-ik). An organism living off another.

*Pavlov's dogs. Dogs which were trained by the great Russian scientist to become physically ready for food before the food actually appeared. For a period of time he would ring a bell before each meal . The dogs eventually secreted saliva in preparation for the food -- even if the food was not forthcoming .

*Precursor. Something which goes before.

*Streptococcus thermophilus (strep-to-cok-us therm-o-fel-is)

*Trichinosis (trik-in-o-sis). A usually mild, but sometimes fatal, disease of the muscles caused by an intestinal round worm .

THINGS TO THINK ABOUT
YOU ARE WHAT YOU EAT!
--I've eaten so many preservatives my stomach should live 1000 years.
--I'm never too busy to put on weight.
--Obesity proves that the Lord does not help those who help themselves. . . and help themselves. . . and help themselves.
--A minute on your lips—forever on your hips!
DIETING
--A diet is a period of starvation which occurs just before we gain 5 pounds.
--Dieting is for people who want to gain weight more slowly.

-- I knew it was time to diet when I wore all white to a party and the hostess showed movies on me.

--It would be much easier to lose weight if the replacement parts were not so readily available -- in the pantry and refrigerator .

--Dieting is the system of starving yourself to death so that you can live longer.

--Dieting takes will power -- there is no substitute for it.

-- Dieting is a system of starving herself to death so that you'll live longer

--"Dieting isn't for everyone. Some people function better when they are fat ." Dr . Hilde Bruche, Processor of Psychiatry, Baylor University.

SENSIBLE EATING

--"Eat not to dullness, drink not to elevation." Benjamin Franklin

--Rule of tum: the more second helpings, the fewer second glances!

--We bought a crock pot because it cooks slow and a microwave oven because it cooks fast.

--If my breakfast coffee is a stimulant why do I sleep through my first class?

HEALTHY ACTION

If you are interested in dieting to lose weight--keep a diary for one week noting the exact time and places that you eat. Note also what you were thinking or doing just prior to eating. This may give you an understanding of the stresses or the cues which have "programmed" you to eat.

Using the Nutritive Value of Foods Guide (available from the U.S. Government Printing Office or online), identify the foods which are high in protein. Identify those which are low in total fats. Identify those which are high in monounsaturated (oleic) and polyunsaturated (linoleic acid) and saturated fats.

Using the Nutritive Value of Foods Guide, compute the intake of your diet on the pages provided on the worksheet. Does your present diet meet the minimum standards listed on the last page of the Nutritive Value of Foods guide?

SOME GLYCEMIC RATINGS—LOW IS BETTER

GRAINS

Pearl barley Low 25 Rye Low 34 Wheat kernels Low 41 Rice, instant Low 46 Rice, parboiled Low 48 Barley, cracked Low 50 Rice, brown Medium 55 Rice, wild Medium 57 Rice, white Medium 58 Barley, flakes Medium 66 Taco Shell Medium 68 Millet High 71

PASTERIES

Pound cake Low 54 Danish pastry Medium 59 Muffin (unsweetened) Medium 62 Cake , tart Medium 65 Cake, angel Medium 67 Croissant Medium 67 Waffles High 76 Doughnut High 76

BISCUITS AND WAFERS

Digestives Medium 58 Shortbread Medium 64 Water biscuits Medium 65 Ryvita Medium 67 Wafer biscuits High 77 Rice cakes High 77

BREADS

Multi grain bread Low 48 Whole grain Low 50 Pita bread, white Medium 57 Pizza, cheese Medium 60 Hamburger bun Medium 61 Rye-flour bread Medium 64 Whole meal bread Medium 69 White bread High 71 White rolls High 73 Baguette High 95

BREAKFAST CEREALS

All-Bran Low 42 Porridge, non instant Low 49 Oat bran Medium 55 Muesli Medium 56 Mini Wheats (wholemeal) Medium 57 Shredded Wheat Medium 69 Golden Grahams High 71 Puffed wheat High 74 Weetabix High 77 Rice Krispies High 82 Cornflakes High 83

PASTA

Spaghetti, protein enriched Low 27 Fettuccine Low 32 Vermicelli Low 35 Spaghetti, whole wheat Low 37 Ravioli, meat filled Low 39 Spaghetti, white Low 41 Macaroni Low 45 Spaghetti, durum wheat Medium 55 Macaroni cheese Medium 64 Rice pasta, brown High 92

DRINKS—FRUIT JUICES AND SOYA

Soya milk Low 30 Apple juice Low 41 Carrot juice Low 45 Pineapple juice Low 46 Grapefruit juice Low 48 Orange juice Low 52

DAIRY

Yogurt low- fat (sweetened) Low 14 Milk, chocolate Low 24 Milk, whole Low 27 Milk, Fat-free Low 32 Milk ,skimmed Low 32 Milk, semi-skimmed Low 34 *Ice-cream (low- fat) Low 50 *Ice-cream Medium 61

FRUITS

Cherries Low 22 Grapefruit Low 25 Apricots (dried) Low 31 Apples Low 38 Pears Low 38 Plums Low 39 Peaches Low 42 Oranges Low 44 Grapes Low 46 Kiwi fruit Low 53 Bananas Low 54 Fruit cocktail Medium 55 Mangoes Medium 56 Apricots Medium 57 Apricots (tinned in syrup) Medium 64 Raisins Medium 64 Pineapple Medium 66 **Watermelon High 72

VEGETABLES AND BEANS

Artichoke Low 15 Asparagus Low 15 Broccoli Low 15 Cauliflower Low 15 Celery Low 15 Cucumber Low 15 Eggplant Low 15 Green beans Low 15 Lettuce, all varieties Low 15 Low-fat yogurt, artificially sweetened Low 15 Peppers, all varieties Low 15 Snow peas Low 15 Spinach Low 15 Young summer squash Low 15 Tomatoes Low 15 Zucchini Low 15 Soya beans, boiled Low 16 Peas, dried Low 22 Kidney beans, boiled Low 29 Lentils green, boiled Low 29 Chickpeas Low 33 Haricot beans, boiled Low 38 Black-eyed beans Low 41 Chickpeas, tinned Low 42 Baked beans, tinned Low 48 Kidney beans, tinned Low 52 Lentils green, tinned Low 52 Broad beans High 79

ROOT VEGETABLES

Carrots, cooked Low 39 Yam Low 51 Sweet potato Low 54 Potato, boiled Medium 56 Potato, new Medium 57 Potato, tinned Medium 61 Beetroot Medium 64 Potato, steamed Medium 65 Potato, mashed Medium 70 Chips High 75 Potato, micro waved High 82 Potato, instant High 83 **Potato, baked High 85 Parsnips High 97

SOUPS

Tomato soup, tinned Low 38 Lentil soup, tinned Low 44 Black bean soup, tinned Medium 64 Green pea soup, tinned Medium 66

SNACK FOOD AND SWEETS

Peanuts Low 15 *M&Ms (peanut) Low 32 *Snickers bar Low 40 *Chocolate bar; 30g Low 49 Jams and marmalades Low 49 *Crisps Low 54 Popcorn Medium 55 Mars bar Medium 64 *Table sugar (sucrose) Medium 65 Corn chips High 74 Jelly beans High 80 Pretzels High 81 Dates High 103

CALORIC EXPENDITURE FOR VARIOUS ACTIVITIES

Inactive way	Kcals used	Active way	Kcals used
Use TV remote	<1	Get up to change channel	3
Phone calls 30 min, reclining	4	Phone calls 30 min, standing	20
Hire home help	0	Iron 30 min, vacuum 30 min	152
Heat up a microwave meal	15	Cook 30 min	25
Buy pre-sliced vegetables	0	Prepare vegetables	10–13
Use leaf blower 30 min	100	Rake leaves 30 min	150
Hire a gardener	0	Garden or mow lawn 30 min	360
Use car wash	18	Wash and wax car 1 hour	300
Let dog out of back door	2	Walk dog 30 min	125
Drive 40 min, walk 5 min	22	Walk 15 min to bus	60
Email a friend, 4 min	2–3	Walk 1 min, stand and talk 3 min	6
Take lift up three floors	0.3	Climb three flights stairs	15
Park at door of supermarket	0.3	Park and walk 2 min	1.6
Watch TV for 1 hour	30	Walk and shop 1 hour	145

Inactive way	Active way
Uses 1,700 kcals per month	Uses 10,500 kcals per month

END NOTES

1. Linda Partridge, Ph.D. Diet and Healthy Aging. N Engl J Med 2012; December 27, 2012. 367:2550-2551

2. Bishop, D. Dietary supplements and team sport performance. Sports Med. 2010 Dec 1;40(12):995-1017.

3. Nutter, J. Seasonal changes in female athletes' diets. International Journal of Sports Nutrition, 1(4) 1991, 395-407.

4.Barrett-Connor, E. "Caffeine and bone fractures," Journal of American Medical Assn. Jan. 26, 1994.

5. Univ. of California Wellness Letter, Jan. 1992, pp 1-2.

6. Los Angeles Times Feb. 3, 1994; Tufts University Nutrition Letter, 12:2, Apr. 1994, p. 1.

7. Briggs, George M. and Calloway, Doris. Bogert's Nutrition and Physical Fitness. Philadelphia: W. B. Saunders. 1979. p. 246.

8. Vudhivai, A. et al. Healthy vegetarians are still shown to be at a higher risk for deficiencies in vitamins B1, B6, B12, and D. Med J Thailand. 1991.

9. Bourn D, Prescott J.. A comparison of the nutritional value, sensory qualities, and food safety of organically and conventionally produced foods Critical Reviews in Food Science Nutrition. Jan 2002: 42(1): 1–34.

10. Manner, T. et al. "Fish oils and the lung." Clinical Nutrition. 12:3, June 1993, p. 131.

11 www.nlm.nih.gov

12. Thomas, Tom. Fitness and Health Promotion. Dubuque: Eddie Bowers. 1993.

13. N Engl J Med. Dec. 2, 2010; 363:2211-2219.

14. Source of basic data Build Study, 1979. Society of Actuaries and Association of Life Insurance Medical Directors of America, 1980. Copyright© 1996, 1999 Metropolitan Life Insurance Company. Courtesy of the Metropolitan Life Insurance Company.

15. Coleman, E. "Nutritional update: dietary carbohydrate and fat and body fat accumulation." Sports Medicine Digest. 10:7, 1988.

16. Report of the National Task Force on the Prevention and Treatment of Obesity, reported in U.S. News and World Report, Oct. 31, 1994 commenting on the journal article in the Journal of the American Medical Association; see also Harvard Health Letter, 3:5, Jan. 1993, p. 2.

17. Goto K, Tanaka K, Ishii N, Uchida S, Takamatsu K. A single versus multiple bouts of moderate-intensity exercise for fat metabolism. Clin Physiol Funct Imaging. 2011 May;31(3):215-20.

18. Hopps E., Caimi G. Exercise in obesity management. J Sports Med Phys Fitness. 2011 Jun;51(2):275-82.

19. Tufts Nutrition Letter, 10:5, July 1992.

20. Larson, TM et al, Diets with High or Low Protein Content and Glycemic Index for Weight-Loss Maintenance. N Engl J Med Nov. 25, 2010; 363:2102-2113.

CHAPTER 10
TOBACCO

R.J. Reynolds III, grandson of the founder of the tobacco company, died in 1994 from two diseases of smoking, emphysema and heart disease. Because of his health problems he gave up smoking in 1988, but it was too late. He was the fifth member of his family to die from smoking related causes. His half brother Patrick conducted a memorial service in Los Angeles. Patrick had long ago sold all of his stocks in the tobacco company and had spent over $2.5 million of his inheritance in anti-smoking causes. (Los Angeles Times July 15, 1994)

If you still smoke—here are some things to think about, -

Cigarette smoking is without a doubt the greatest single public health problem the West has ever faced. In 1964, the Surgeon General of the United States reported to the nation that cigarettes were definitely causative of lung cancer and many other lung diseases. That slowed up a few smokers, but the health risks of smoking keep mounting. A British study examining many of the causes of death found that the lowest risk was among those who had never smoked and those who gave up smoking. (Shaper, AG. "Body weight: implications for the prevention of coronary heart disease, stroke, and diabetes mellitus in a cohort study of middle aged men." Brit Med. Jour. May 1997 314 p. 1311)

Tobacco use, not heart disease or cancer, is the number one killer of people in the Western world. (McGinnis, J. Michael. "Actual causes of death in the United States" Journal of American Medical Assn. 270:18513, November 10, 1993. p.p. 2207-12) This study looked at the environmental causes of death not the actual disease from which the person died. Tobacco use was found to cause 400,000 deaths for the year of 1990. Poor diet and lack of exercise together accounted for 300,000 deaths The diseases which actually caused the physical death were: heart disease, cancers, strokes, and low birth weights of the babies of smoking mothers. Together these accounted for 19% of all deaths in the United States.

THE INGREDIENTS OF CIGARETTE SMOKE

In every balanced blend of fine aromas in cigarette smoke, there are more than 4000 different chemicals, 40 have been proven to be carcinogenic. (1) Among these are acids, aldehydes, ketones, hydrocarbons, arsenic, carbon monoxide, nitrogen dioxide, nicotine, cancer producing agents, ammonia, nitric oxide, benzene, hydrocyanic acid, and tars. Tars carry these cancer producing agents. The one-pack-a-day smoker inhales about eight ounces (a half of a pint of tar solids) into the lungs each year. At least 60 per cent of the "country fresh flavor" which is inhaled in every puff of smoke is therefore relatively deadly.

There is some evidence that smoking low-tar, low nicotine cigarettes can reduce the amount of tar in the lungs. An American Cancer Society report showed deaths from lung cancer were 26 per cent less among the low-tar cigarette smokers than among the high-tar cigarette smokers. Death from heart disease was 14 per cent less for the low-tar smokers. Other findings were that deaths from lung cancer for non-smokers were only 15 per cent of that for low-tar smokers. So low tar smokers die from lung cancer about seven times more often than the non-smokers.

Nicotine is a fast acting poison which is sometimes used in insecticides. Its effects on the body include: the mobilizing of fatty acids, which increases the cholesterol level of the blood; the constricting of blood vessels in the skin, which increases blood pressure; and the stimulation, then the depression, of the nervous system. As is now known, nicotine is highly addictive--second only to cocaine and its derivatives.

The lethal adult dose is 60 milligrams. Depending on the brand, a cigarette contains 0.05 to 2.5 milligrams, averaging under 1%, of which 80 to 90% reaches the bloodstream. A cigar contains 120 milligrams (double the lethal dose) but a non-inhaling cigar smoker takes in only 20 to 50% of the available nicotine. (2)

Nicotine is metabolized in the liver. The metabolism takes about 25 minutes to break down half of the nicotine present. (This is called a half-life.) By the time the nicotine has been reduced to 30 to 50% of the original dosage, the addicted smoker needs another dose.

Arsenic is a lethal poison. It has been greatly reduced in cigarettes during the last 15 years, yet the average smoker takes 40 to 50 milligrams per day; 20 per cent of this is still present in the body after four days. It has an accumulative buildup. Arsenic in smoke has produced cancer in mice.

Benzene is a highly toxic substance. In 1990 the Food and Drug Administration forced a recall of a famous mineral water because it was contaminated with benzene. A cigarette has about 2000 times more benzene in it than did a bottle of that water. Benzene is also prohibited to be used in the manufacture of several compounds, including paint thinner.

Benzopyrine is a carcinogenic agent found in both tobacco and marijuana. Its exact role in the human cancer process is not yet known but studies of mice have shown cancer in both the adults and the babies of mice who were exposed to the substance.

Nitrogen dioxide (NO_2) is considered hazardous in air pollution when it reaches five parts per million. In cigarette smoke, it is 250 parts per million.

Carbon monoxide exposure of 120 parts per million for one hour can cause dizziness, headache, and exhaustion. Cigarette smoke contains 42, 000 parts per million.

Hydrogen cyanide works against respiratory enzymes. Long-term exposure above 10 parts per million is dangerous. Cigarette smoke contains 1600 parts per million.

Ammonia is added to cigarettes to preserve and maintain the nicotine level.

IMMEDIATE EFFECTS OF SMOKING ON THE BODY

As soon as one takes a few puffs from a cigarette, the central nervous system is stimulated by nicotine. Nicotine first acts as a stimulant, then after it wears off the effect on the body is that of a depressant. This increases the need for another cigarette to re-stimulate the body. At the same time nicotine acts like the neurotransmitter acetylcholine in the synapse of the nerves. This gives a calming effect. So cigarettes give both an upper and a downer effect at the same time. It is the only drug that gives two such strong actions simultaneously. This is why the withdrawal from nicotine is so difficult. The addicted person withdraws with an upper reaction, as in a heroin withdrawal, from the depressant effects of not having the drug. Simultaneously there is a crashing reaction, somewhat similar to that from cocaine, from the stimulant effects of the drug. While neither reaction is as strong as a withdrawal from heroin or cocaine, the combination withdrawal makes it very difficult to overcome. This is why withdrawal from nicotine is considered the third most difficult drug from which to withdraw--after crack cocaine and regular cocaine.

As noted, nicotine, which is found exclusively in tobacco, increases the adrenaline and adrenaline-like substances, which in turn increase blood pressure. This can be dangerous to anybody who has a tendency toward stroke or heart disease. It speeds up the heart rate by as much as 20 beats per minute. It therefore increases the need for oxygen in the heart. However because of the increased carbon monoxide in the blood there is not sufficient oxygen for the heart's increased needs. This is believed to be a factor in the increased number of heart attacks among smokers. It also releases fats into the blood, especially cholesterol, so that the cholesterol level of the blood is raised. This increases the hardening of the arteries.

Hunger and the desire for food are generally reduced. Nicotine raises the blood sugar level, one of the things that gives people the feeling of energy. It also inhibits stomach contractions. In addition it numbs the taste buds so food doesn't taste as good.

It also shortens the blood clotting time. In fact, one cigarette can hasten the blood clotting time by as much as 25 per cent. This effect lasts from 15 minutes to 3 hours and is probably a prime reason for the increased heart attack rate in smokers. There is also a constriction of the arteries of the heart so that a smaller blood clot can block the blood flow..

Additionally there is an effect on the respiratory system. Smoking constricts the bronchial tubes which reduces the amount of air which can reach the lungs. Just one cigarette damages the lungs. It paralyzes the cilia (hair-like organs) which carry dirt and other foreign substances from the lungs back to the nose and the mouth. In heavy smokers, the cilia have entirely disappeared.

The smoker's cough in the morning is due to the fact that the small hairs in the breathing passages, which have been anesthetized by the smoke, begin to come alive again. Their movements and the increased mucus, which is also developed by the smoking, tickles and irritates the breathing passages and causes the smoker to cough. This increase in mucus becomes a breeding ground for germs, possibly accounting for the increased number of colds in smokers.

Smoking also narrows the visual field and impairs a person's ability to drive at night. It also decreases athletic performance, especially in the endurance sports which require great stamina such as swimming, distance running, soccer and basketball.

Carbon monoxide is a very dangerous element in cigarette smoke. It combines with the hemoglobin, the iron compound in the red blood cells which transports the oxygen from the lungs to the cells. But since the hemoglobin has 200 times more affinity for the carbon monoxide than it does for oxygen, the carbon monoxide can starve out the oxygen, which is necessary to live. Carbon monoxide then becomes a poison because the oxygen in the carbon monoxide cannot be released to the cells. This makes the blood less efficient. As much as 10% of a smoker's red blood cells can be made useless because they are carrying carbon monoxide rather than oxygen. (3) Any increase in carbon monoxide makes the heart pump faster since more blood is needed to bring the necessary oxygen to the tissues. Carbon monoxide in cigarettes is 640 times greater than the level considered safe for industrial plants.

People who commit suicide by locking themselves in a garage and turning on the car engine die because the carbon monoxide in the car exhaust starves out the oxygen in the blood. When an excess of the gas is absorbed into the blood, a coma begins--and death will follow shortly as the percentage of carbon monoxide increases in the blood and starves the body's organs of the needed oxygen.

The carbon monoxide in cigarette smoke can impair eyesight, manual dexterity, reflexes, and the ability to estimate time intervals. These effects are worsened at higher altitudes. Because of the effects of carbon monoxide, the average smoker at sea level gets about the same efficiency from his lungs as does a non-smoker living at an altitude of 8, 000 feet above sea level

A study done by the Environmental Protection Agency covering 29, 000 people in 18 metropolitan areas showed the effects of pollution and smoking on the carbon monoxide level of the blood. Suburban non-smokers showed from 0. 4 to 1. 5 per cent carbon monoxide in the blood. City-living non-smokers ranged from 0. 8 to 3. 2, averaging 1. 5 per cent in their blood. Most of the nonsmokers in Los Angeles, Denver, Chicago, and San Francisco exceeded that 1.5 average of carbon monoxide in the blood. If these people smoked, it added another four per cent to the carbon monoxide level, so Los Angeles smokers averaged 6. 2 per cent carbon monoxide, and some people measured over 10 per cent of blood carbon monoxide. Smokers with serious cardiovascular problems have their powers seriously impaired when their carbon monoxide level is over 3. 5 per cent.

Smoking even one cigarette interrupts the body's production of collagen for 30 to 40 minutes. Collagen is a substance which is used to mend broken bones and other wounds. So smoking slows the healing process. This is a result of the reduced oxygen in the blood due to smoking. Collagen breakdown also causes wrinkles in the skin.

Smoking also reduces fertility in men and may increase impotency (inability to achieve an erection) both occur because of low oxygen in the blood and a reduction of male hormones. Both are quickly reversible after stopping smoking. Female hormones are also reduced. This can cause menstrual irregularities, infertility, and the growth of facial hair.

THE LONG-TERM EFFECTS OF SMOKING

Smoking increases the death rate to a great degree. It hardens the arteries; doubles the heart attack rate; increases the emphysema rate by four to six times; and increases the lung cancer rate by 8 or more times. It also increases the chances of many other diseases. Smokers arrive at old age with 20 to 30% less bone density and with more risk of fractures, than do non-smokers. In the case of AIDS, it doubles the speed at which the symptoms develop. (4)

In the age group forty-five to sixty-four, non-smokers die at the rate of 708 persons per 100, 000 population. Smokers die at the rate of 1329 persons per 100, 000 population. Of these, heart disease accounts for 615 of the smokers' deaths but only 304 of the non-smokers' deaths. Lung cancer accounts for 87 deaths for the smokers and 11 for the non-smokers. Emphysema accounts for 24 of the smokers' deaths and 4 of the non-smokers' deaths.

There are various estimates as to how much smoking shortens a life. For a teenager, it probably shortens life about eight to fourteen years. However, official statistics compiled in Germany indicate that the non-smoker lives seven years longer than the average smoker of one pack a day and 14 years longer than the chain smoker. Recent studies indicate that a 35 year old man who smokes two packs a day reduces his life expectancy by more than 8 years. (5)

Studies on the average increase of death rates for smokers are difficult to compare because it is generally not known exactly when each smoker started to smoke, what percentage of cigarettes were high tar and nicotine or low tar and nicotine, exactly how many cigarettes were smoked, and how much side stream (passive smoke) was inhaled by the smokers and the non-smokers in the study. Hereditary weaknesses of the participants in the study is also a factor. The one fact is clear--that smoking greatly decreases the life expectancy of the average smoker.

Clearly smoking ages the smoker. It shows in the aging of the skin and even the graying of one's hair. (6)

It also increases the risk of hip fractures due to osteoporosis. The estimated cumulative risk of hip fracture in women in England was 19% in smokers and 12% in non-smokers to age 85; 37% and 22% to age 90. Among all women, one hip fracture in eight is attributable to smoking. Limited data in men suggest a similar proportionate effect of smoking as in women.

Cigarettes kill most of their victims through heart attacks. Lung cancer claims the second greatest number, and emphysema is third. It is widely believed that smoking 200, 000 cigarettes (a pack a day for 25 years) is almost certain to cause one's death through lung cancer, heart attack, or by some other means. A recent New York study on women and smoking showed that for women dying of coronary heart disease (heart attacks), the average age for death for non-smokers was 67 years, for light smokers it was 55 years, and for heavy smokers, 48 years.

Since two of the major factors associated with higher death risk, nicotine and tars, can be found in differing amounts in different brands of cigarettes smokers of low tar, low nicotine cigarettes can reduce the expected death rate by 15 to 20% of the rates of the average smoker. However the carbon monoxide inhaled from any cigarette is approximately the same--and it is a highly damaging element to have in the blood.

Atherosclerosis (hardened arteries) in monkeys and rabbits was increased when they breathed increased carbon monoxide for 15 minutes a day for a year. Animal studies show that carbon monoxide makes the artery walls more permeable to fatty substances. This is one likely possibility to help to explain the high heart attack rate among smokers. Possibly more important, smoking increases the amount of cholesterol in the blood and it also reduces the amount of HDL (the good cholesterol) which thereby increases the amount of artery hardening and clogging.

Many cancers are increased by smoking. Leukemia, a blood cancer, is increased by 30% (3,600 cases). (Archives of Internal Medicine, Feb. 1993, reported in University of California Wellness Letter, Vol. 9 (8) May 1993, p. 1) In fact 30% of all cancers are caused by smoking. (American Cancer Society--Cancer Response System, number 252. Sept. 1, 1992)

Other cancer risks are also increased: bladder cancer (40% increase), cervical cancer, esophageal cancer (80% of all cases), cancers of the stomach and colon (double the risk of non-smokers), laryngeal cancer (25 times more), kidney cancers (40% of all cases), mouth cancer (27 times higher), breast cancer (75%.)

Lung Cancer caused only one death in 500 in the year 1890. Today the rate is one in 14. This increase is due mostly to smoking cigarettes. Since there are 50, 000 times more particles in cigarette smoke than in heavy air pollution, it is easy to understand how hard it is for the lungs and the bronchial tubes to try to clean themselves of these particles.

We assume that, based on studies, cigarettes are more harmful than pipes in lung cancer. This was reported by the American Cancer Society. However, a recent Swedish study which dealt with 27, 000 men and an equal number of women aged eighteen to sixty-nine showed that the lung cancer rates for cigarette and pipe smokers were about even. They each had seven times more lung cancer than did non-smokers. And those who smoked both cigarettes and pipes had 11 times the risk. In fact, pipe smokers who consumed as many as 15 cigarettes a day showed 29 times the risk of lung cancer. The difference may be due to the type of tobacco used and whether the pipe smokers inhaled.

Non-inhaling smokers, such as pipe and cigar smokers, tend to develop cancers of the mouth, larynx, esophagus, and on the tongue and lips. Inhalers tend to develop cancers of the lungs, the bladder, and the pancreas. Lung cancer, once it has developed, is 90 per cent fatal.

Seventh Day Adventist Church, which does not allow its members to smoke, has a very low lung cancer rate among its members, even when they live in cities where there is a great deal of air pollution. On the other hand, the people in Iceland, where there is very little air pollution and a high percentage of cigarette smokers, have a high rate of lung cancer. Statistics indicate that if you stop smoking for 10 years, your chances of getting lung cancer are no greater than that of the non-smoker.

Emphysema and chronic bronchitis each year are increased by about a million new cases. Most of them are brought on by smoking. It is estimated that 99 per cent of heavy cigarette smokers (smokers who smoke more than a pack a day) have emphysema. In a study of 1800 deceased people, only 10 per cent of the non-smokers had any degree of emphysema, and none had advanced emphysema.

In chronic smokers, the increased mucus in the bronchial tubes can drop into the lungs and have the same effect as water in the lungs, in effect "drowning" the smoker because the mucus-filled alveoli (air sacs in the lungs) are not able to accept oxygen. This is caused not only by the increased mucus but also by the loss of the cilia which would be able to eliminate some of the mucus.

Other problems include:

--Back pain, a common ailment among smokers and the leading cause of worker disability. The poor oxygen levels in the blood prevent the lumbar discs from being adequately oxygenated.

--The chance of getting stomach ulcers. The levels of prostaglandins, which help to protect the stomach lining, is reduced. Estimates are that there are a million more ulcers per year because of smoking.

--Increased risk of: stroke (twice to six times the risk--depending on amount smoked).

--Increased diabetes risk.

--Osteoporosis in women (five times greater).

--Premature aging of the skin.

--Yellowing of teeth and fingernails, .

--More of the mouth and gums diseases. Female smokers, aged twenty to thirty-nine, and male smokers, aged thirty to fifty-nine, have twice the chances of being completely toothless from periodontal diseases than do non-smokers.

--More colds.

--More cirrhosis of the liver. The cirrhosis may be because smokers often drink more alcohol, and the disease may be due more to the drinking and the lack of food than with the effects of smoking.

--Blindness (nicotine amblyopia) may result from the nicotine in tobacco. This is especially true for cigar and pipe smokers.

Smoking also seems to dull one's sex life, possibly because nicotine poisons the central nervous system, and possibly because it interferes with the male hormone secretion. It also seems to affect male fertility. It reduces the sperm production and may change the structural quality of the sperm. A recent study reported by the Soviet Newspaper, Soviet Skaya Rossiya, reported that scientists have just completed a study showing that smoking causes chemical changes in the blood in the sex hormones. Men over forty were most seriously affected.

GIVING UP SMOKING

Many millions of people have given up smoking. The obvious health reasons seem to be the primary motivation for giving up smoking. Before giving up smoking, it is a good idea to determine the type of smoker you are. Four types of smokers have been identified:

1. About 50 per cent smoke for "positive effect." This smoker wants a cigarette when he or she is most relaxed, such as after a meal or while drinking coffee or liquor. To quit, this smoker should find another pleasant habit to substitute for his or her smoking. This smoker's chances of quitting are good.

2. About 40 per cent smoke for "negative effect. " They use smoking as a crutch--to delay doing unpleasant tasks. They smoke when ill at ease, frustrated, or nervous. If they give up smoking, they are most likely to begin again if tense situations develop.

3. Ten per cent of smokers are "habitual" smokers. They smoke without thinking about it, without really enjoying it. These people find it easiest to quit. They need only be reconditioned not to smoke.

4. About 35 per cent of smokers are "addicted. " (Some people are in more than one of the above categories.) This person feels unhappy when not able to smoke. Going without a cigarette can be intolerable. For this person to quit it must be done "cold turkey."

There are three stages in giving up smoking.

1. Contemplation. First you must think about why you want to give up the habit. How strong is your motivation? You may have begun to think of quitting because of your increased knowledge about the many negative effects of smoking. But this may not have changed your attitude sufficiently yet. You will need a strong commitment to quitting because nicotine is an extremely addictive drug. If you do find that you have a sufficiently strong motivation you can honestly decide to quit.

2. Quitting . There are many approaches to quitting. Some people stop by themselves, some use nicotine patches, some use educational and self help groups. The actual difficulty with quitting is dependent on how heavily you are addicted to nicotine. If you try but fail to quit you may be comforted to know that your chances of finally quitting increase with each attempt.

3. Maintenance. Staying nicotine free gets easier with each passing week. During this time avoid the temptation of "just one smoke." It is so easy to relapse. Also, during the early stages of your quitting ask friends and family not to smoke in your presence--or leave when they light up

If you have been a very heavy smoker and you decide to give up smoking, you may exhibit withdrawal symptoms from the depressant effects. Such effects can include: chattering teeth, uncontrollable shakes, and chilling. The results of withdrawing from the stimulant effects of the release of adrenaline and norepinephrine can include depression. These usually begin within three hours and if they occur, they will be during the first day of not smoking. During this time poisons, which have been built up by smoking, begin to affect the body. It takes between three weeks and three months for them to be totally released by the body. There will often be other discomforts such as a lack of efficiency and tenseness during the time that you are giving up smoking.

There is no magic way to give up smoking by which a person will not experience some discomfort. Here are some suggestions for methods you might use to stop the smoking habit.

--Since the major problem in giving up smoking is the withdrawal from the potent chemical nicotine, it has been found that nicotine replacement methods (such as gum, lozenges, and skin patches) work best. Each of these methods is about 30% effective in helping a person to quit.

--Behavior modification should help in working on the psychological reasons for smoking. You might try any or all of the following techniques:

--Do something whenever you feel the urge to smoke. You might chew gum or exercise. Try a 20-minute walk after dinner. This not only helps to keep you a little better fit, but it also keeps you occupied at a time when you would normally be smoking.

-- Don't let yourself get angry or hungry.

--Briskly rub your body with a warm washcloth to counteract the chronic vaso-constriction of the blood vessels of the skin.

--Drink at least six to eight glasses of water or juices a day. Cranberry juice is particularly good. This facilitates the excretion of nicotine and its byproducts. The high intake of fruit and fruit juices is desirable because acid urine aids in nicotine excretion. Fruit sugars also help the ex-smoker to tolerate the drop in blood sugar which occurs after nicotine withdrawal. Dried fruits can be eaten when there is a craving for a cigarette.

--One should not drink alcohol for the first five days of smoking abstinence because it might lessen one's determination to stop smoking. If you need to relax, you might try deep breathing exercises or other stress management techniques. These may help to relieve any withdrawal anxieties.

--Coffee also increases the withdrawal symptoms from the nicotine so coffee drinking should be curbed during nicotine withdrawal.

Hypnosis has been successfully used by some smokers. While this method has not been studied extensively, early reports indicate that it may have a success rate of between 25 and 40% for the first two year period.

If you cannot stop smoking, you might consider using filters or smoking each cigarette less since the last part of the cigarette is the most harmful. The tobacco in the cigarette assists in filtering out some of the harmful substances, but when you smoke the last part of the cigarette you are taking in those harmful substances from the first several puffs which had been trapped on the tobacco closer to the smoker's lips.

Some people have tried to cut down their tar and nicotine intake by changing to low tar, low nicotine cigarettes. Some use these cigarettes as they try to taper off and eventually quit their habits. Others want to continue to smoke, but want to lessen the negative effects on their bodies. But if they are smoking to get the effect of the nicotine they will probably smoke more cigarettes. This is probably why the average smoker today smokes more cigarettes than did the average smoker of 1955, when high nicotine brands were popular. One reason for smoking more cigarettes is that there is less tobacco in cigarettes today than there was 25 years ago. The amount of tobacco required to make 1, 000 cigarettes today is only 1. 9 pounds compared with the 2.7 pounds used a quarter of a century ago.

Many people find that the most effective way to quit smoking is to attend a stop-smoking clinic. Most are very reasonably priced.

SELF TEST

1. Nicotine is the most dangerous element in tobacco smoke. ___

2. Nicotine is an addictive substance which is not much more addictive than the caffeine in coffee. _____

3. The taxes on cigarettes pay all of the medical costs which smoking causes. ____

4. Sidestream smoke inhaled by those near the smoker is less dangerous than the smoke which the smoker inhales. ____

5. The illnesses caused by smokers cost the taxpayers nearly a billion dollars per year in medical bills. ____

6. The major cause of death for smokers is lung cancer. ____

7. Smokeless tobacco is a safe way of using tobacco. ____

8. Every year fewer Americans are smoking. ____

9. Teenage girls take up the smoking habit more often than any other group. ____

10. Stop smoking clinics generally work. ____

ANSWERS

1. T or F. While nicotine is the addictive agent in tobacco smoke, the tars, carbon monoxide, or any of a number of other compounds may actually be more dangerous.

2. F Nicotine is highly addictive, ranking close behind crack cocaine and cocaine but more addictive than heroin.

3. F Only a minor percentage of the medical costs are covered by taxes.

4. T or F Since the sidestream smoke is not filtered it is more dangerous as it comes off the cigarette, but because it is not as concentrated when it reaches the nose of the passive smoker it is less dangerous at that point.

5. F Non-smokers pay over $22 billion dollars a year for the illnesses of smokers.

6. F Far more smokers die of tobacco related heart disease than lung cancer.

7. F A number of cancers are caused by smokeless tobacco.

8. From 1968 until the early 1990's smoking decreased. It has now leveled off.

9. T

10. F No technique has been developed which helps smokers to stop in a high percentage of cases. However, the more often a smoker attempts to stop the better the chances are of success. So while clinics work for a few the first time, they work progressively more often with each new attempt by a smoker to stop.

END NOTES

American Cancer Society-Cancer Response System, No. 2522, Dec. 23, 1993

Jaffe, J.H. "Drug addiction and drug abuse" in The Pharmacological Basis of Therapeutics, A.G. Gilman (ed), 6th edit. New York: Macmillan, 1980; U.S. Surgeon General. The Changing Cigarette. Publication no. 81-51056. Washington, D.C. Dept. of Health, Education, and Welfare. 1981; Volle, R.L. and Koelle, G.B. "Ganglionic stimulating and blocking agents," in Gilman, op.cit. 1975) Tobacco companies have been able to raise a type of tobacco which has a nicotine level of 6%. This is illegal to grow in the United States . (FDA report cited in Los Angeles Times, July 18, 1994, p A 12)

Palfai, T. and Jankiewicz, H. Drugs and Human Behavior. Dubuque, IA: Wm. C. Brown, 1991

Neiman, Richard. Aids and Smoking. AIDS, May 1993)

U.S. Surgeon General. The Health Consequences of Smoking. Washington, D.C. Government Printing Office, 1985.

Bulpitt C J, Shipley M J, Broughton P M G,Fletcher A E, Markowe H L J, Marmot M G, et al. The assessment of biological age. (Ageing Clin Exp Res. 1994; 6:181-91.)

CHAPTER 11
ILLEGAL DRUGS AND ALCOHOL

Our attempts to change reality chemically

In November 2012 the California Office of Traffic Safety conducted a study analyzing the breath of about 1500 drivers. They found that one in seven was high on some type of drug, legal or illegal, and one in 14 were high on alcohol. If you want to live a long life you must be aware that drugs can impair your driving and possibly lead to an injury or death. But also you need to be aware that about one in five drivers may be driving impaired. You therefore need to drive defensively because not everybody is as sober as you are.

For your own information, and for information you may want to pass on, we will discuss drugs in general, then alcohol.

People take psychoactive drugs to forget their problems, to reduce inhibitions, or to get pleasure. These goals are accomplished by changing the electrical action in different parts of the brain. So it is not far-fetched to think that in the future actual electricity might be used rather than using chemicals to change the brain's electrical circuitry as is done today.

HISTORY OF DRUG USE

Altering behavior has been a continuous goal of humankind throughout recorded history. The Egyptians are given credit for the first brewery. It dates back to 3700 B.C. They are also given credit for the first written lessons regarding the evils of alcohol. That appeared about

3,000 years ago. In India about 4,000 years ago a holy drug called Soma was noted. It is not certain whether this was alcohol, marijuana, or a stimulant called ephedrine.

In 2737 B. C. the Chinese emperor Shen Nung wrote a book about drugs. He accurately described the effects of smoking the cannabis plant. About 2,000 years later, while the Chinese government was attempting to establish a monopoly for wine making, another emperor wrote about the harmful effects of wine.

The holy men in the ancient Hindu religion use a self-induced mental state in order to alter consciousness and become one with God. This is called meditation. It usually takes years to accomplish. Recent new techniques, which purport to do the same thing in much less time, have been developed. The Maharishi Mahesh Yogi has publicized his ideas for relaxing through Transcendental Meditation. Psychologists have worked with biofeedback to assist people in reaching the restful "alpha wave" state. This is the brain wave pattern which yogi's show when they report being "one with God".

So altering the human state of consciousness to escape the realities of the human predicament is not a recent phenomenon. Drugging, especially by using alcohol or marijuana, is apparently at least as old as recorded history. And warnings against such drugging also appear in the early recorded history of the race. The leaders of human societies have long observed the negative effects of an individual's use of drugs on the well-being of the whole of society.

PSYCHOACTIVE DRUGS AND THE BRAIN

Psychoactive means "acting on the psyche." Not all drugs act on the brain. Cortisone is a steroid that works on inflammations in many parts of the body. It reduces pain. Other steroids work primarily in the muscles, making them larger. But they can also affect the brain making people more aggressive. Antibiotics work to kill bacteria in any area of the body. But psychoactive drugs, such as alcohol, marijuana, and cocaine, are used because of their effects on the brain. They do this by changing the normal action of the nerve cells by making them work faster or slower than normal. The effects of the different drugs vary depending on which areas of the brain they affect and whether they increase or decrease the normal electrical activity in that area.

Psychologists have used both drugs and electricity to alter consciousness. Dr. Jose Delgado of Yale implanted electrodes in a fighting bull and was able to control the behavior of the bull. He walked into the bull ring holding a small radio transmitter. When he pushed one button the bull would charge him. Then he would push another button and the bull's rage would be inhibited. It would stop the charge, then walk away.

Electrical stimulation of the hunger control section of the brain can make animals eat so much that they die or starve themselves to death. But James Olds of McGill University may have discovered the ultimate in electrical stimulation of the brain when he accidentally found a "pleasure center" in the brain of a rat. When the rat was allowed to self administer himself with electricity. He liked it. Dr. Olds decided to see how strong that desire was so he put the rat on one side of an electrically charged plate which would be very uncomfortable for the rat if it walked on it. First he starved the rat and put food on

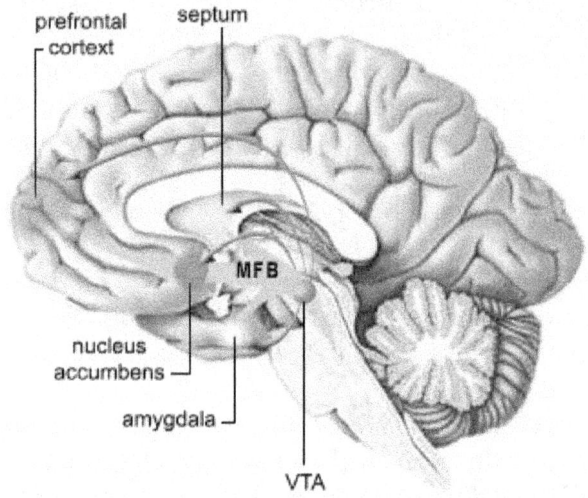

the other side of the electric grid. The rat refused to go over the grid. He preferred to starve to death rather than endure the pain of the grid. However, when Dr. Olds showed that rat that it could get its pleasure center (the medial forebrain bundle) stimulated, the rat crossed the grid. So we might infer that the drive to stimulate the pleasure center is, at least sometimes, greater than the drive for food. No wonder it is so difficult to give up the habits of some drugs--especially those that stimulate the pleasure center.

The continued research into the workings of these deep areas of the human brain has uncovered related areas that are also involved in controlling pleasure or influencing depression. The nucleus accumbens (ACC), the ventral tegmental area (VTA), the lateral hypothalamus and other small interconnected groups of neurons are sometimes separated in the writings of researchers, and sometimes the smaller interconnected areas are included under the general category of the medial forebrain bundle (MFB). These areas have long been known to be influenced by drugs, such as cocaine, amphetamines and the opiates. The electrical pathways between areas are primarily stimulated by dopamine. Many of the psychoactive drugs either increase dopamine, mimic it, or prevent its re-uptake so that it lasts longer in the synapses and has a more long-lasting effect.

More recently these same neural pathways have been found to be related to Parkinson's disease, schizophrenia, attention deficit hyperactivity disorder (ADHD) and to depression. Research in Germany and the US has found that much depression can be reduced or eliminated by electrically stimulating this area. (1) In many cases a single electrical stimulation of the area elicits a long-term or permanent cure of depression.

The point is that our brains work with a combination of electrical impulses and chemicals, called neurotransmitters, and these can be affected by both electrical stimulation and by chemicals, such as the psychoactive drugs. Depending on where the brain is stimulated, chemically or electrically, a person may exhibit depression, hallucinations, intense pleasure, a reduction in pain, a feeling of deep spirituality, or a number of other sensations. We might mention that there are parts of the brain that when stimulated electrically or chemically elicit pain. Obviously nobody takes these drugs recreationally!

As examples of the different areas of the brain that the various drugs affect:

Cocaine and amphetamines activate the release of dopamine in the nucleus accumbens and amygdala through direct actions on dopamine terminals.

Opioids activate opioid receptors in the VTA, nucleus accumbens, and amygdala through direct or indirect actions via interneurons. Opioids facilitate the release of dopamine in the nucleus accumbens by an action either in the VTA or the nucleus accumbens, but also are hypothesized to activate elements independent of the dopamine system.

Alcohol activates another neurotransmitter, GABA. This might be done in the VTA, nucleus accumbens, and amygdala by either direct actions at the GABA receptor or through indirect release of GABA. Alcohol may also directly release opiate-like substances, or some people these substances are result of the breakdown of alcohol in the liver. These opiate like substances can affect the VTA, the nucleus accumbens, and central nucleus of the amygdala. Alcohol facilitates the release of dopamine the nucleus accumbens through an action either in the VTA or the nucleus accumbens.

Nicotine activates nicotinic acetylcholine receptors in the VTA, nucleus accumbens, and amygdala, either directly or indirectly.

Cannabinoids activate cannabinoid CB1 receptors in the VTA, nucleus accumbens, and amygdala. Cannabinoids facilitate the release of dopamine in the nucleus accumbens through an unknown mechanism either in the VTA or the nucleus accumbens.

As you may begin to see, the brain and its workings are extremely complicated. While neuroscientists are studying the many types of brain structures, the different types of neurons, and the ways that these neurons can be stimulated, they are merely scratching the surface at this time. Then there are individual differences between each of us. So, for example, while in the VTA structure tends to have over 50% of neurons that react to dopamine and a large percent that react to GABA, how do you vary from that norm? Do you have a low percent of neurons that react to dopamine? If so might that mean that marijuana does not give you the same effect as it does for a person with a high level of dopamine receptors?.

Endorphins, short for "endogenous morphines" are chemicals (opioid peptides) found in the brain and other parts of the body. They are chemically similar to the opiates (heroin, morphine, etc.) and, like the opiates, make us feel good. There are over 50 such chemicals found so far. They range from being 20 times to several hundred times more powerful per molecule than heroin. The brain has a great number of endorphin receptors. It at these sites that heroin works. Without these receptors opium and its derivatives would not be psychoactive.

Endorphins are released as a response to many events in the brain and body. Classical music releases them. Loud rock music doesn't. Endurance exercise releases them--usually after about 40 minutes of hard exercise. (This is the so called "runner's high.") Pregnancy and labor also increase the amount of endorphins released. This gives the birthing mother a greater resistance to the pain of childbirth. Laughing releases endorphins, as does eating fats and proteins.

The placebo effect is an often noticed effect of research in which the subject gets a feeling or relief merely because it was expected. When a group of people with headaches is given a sugar pill (a placebo), and are told that it is a powerful pain relieving drug, half will get the relief they expected even though there is no chemical reason for the relief. This placebo effect is generally, if not always, the result of endorphins.

An opioid blocker, naloxone, is often given to heroin addicts to stop them from getting the effect of heroin. The same chemical has been found to block the effect of endorphins. In other studies it has been found to block the effect of a placebo

People often want to change their immediate feelings and venture into another type of experience. Small children may make themselves dizzy by spinning around, or see if they can balance themselves while walking on a narrow wall. Teenagers may seek the thrills of an amusement park--the roller coaster, bumper cars, or high speed spinning in giant wheels. Adults may find that their feelings are more complicated and varied so may search for ways to meet their perceived needs--to sleep, to wake up, to feel pleasure, to thrill to a new experience. Drugs are one way, a very simple way, to satisfy these needs.

Another reason people turn to drugs is the effective advertising for the "so-called" positive effects the drugs have. We are constantly being bombarded with pharmaceutical advertisements. Are energy drinks safe? Can I have a better sex life by taking this pill? Will I perform better at work because this pill keeps me from being depressed?

A psycho-active (psychotrophic) drug is any chemical which, if taken in small amounts, can do any of the following: 1) distort one's perceptions, 2) eliminate one's pain, 3) change one's ability to understand information, 4) change a person's mood or emotion, 5) change one's brain wave activity, 6) change a person's physical status such as coordination, consciousness, or activity level.

In earlier days people looked to nature for their drugs--fermenting a grape, chewing a coca leaf, ingesting a mushroom. As science has advanced, it has improved and refined the natural drugs: distilling high proof alcohol from grains, making cocaine and crack from the coca leaf, and making codeine and morphine from opium. More recently it has developed a mass of synthetic drugs which can kill pain, tranquilize, stimulate, and pacify.

Drugs that kill pain, suppress the coughing impulse, lower blood pressure, or relieve depression are welcomed by some in society. But pills, drinks, or injections may make the user a menace to society. For example, the driver under the influence of marijuana or alcohol, the drugged person who totally withdraws from societal responsibilities, or the addict who steals to support a habit, have very negative effects both on themselves and on the society. As you probably know, more people die from prescription drug overdoses than from illegal; drugs. The CDC (Center for Disease Control) has noted an alarming increase in prescription drug deaths since 2003. Nearly 30,000 unintentional prescription drug deaths in 2012, mostly caused by synthetic opioids such as oxycodone. Accidental prescription drug deaths now total more than the total of cocaine and heroin deaths. The temptation to chemically reduce pain as we age should be well considered before popping the pill.

This might be of interest to you—or to your children. Scientists at the United States National Aeronautics and Space Administration (NASA) have turned their attention from the mysteries of the cosmos to a more esoteric area of research: what happens when you get a spider stoned. Their experiments have shown that common house spiders spin their webs in different ways according to the psychotropic drug they have been given. NASA scientists believe the research demonstrates that web-spinning spiders can be used to test drugs because the more toxic the chemical, the more deformed was the web.

Spiders on marijuana appeared to lose concentration about half-way through the spin.

Those on Benzedrine, an upper such as meth (speed) spun their webs fast, but without adequate planning.

Caffeine also seemed to affect planning. Caffeine one of the most common drugs consumed by us in soft drinks, tea and coffee, makes spiders incapable of spinning anything better than a few threads strung together at random.

On chloral hydrate web spinning quit early.

Other research with spiders has turned up some interesting drug related behavior.

--Spiders on certain hallucinatory drugs wove webs with the strands far apart. The spiders apparently felt that they were bigger than they actually were. Researchers concluded that they had delusions of grandeur.

--Spiders given the blood of schizophrenic patients spun bizarre webs. If the blood was drawn when the patient was in a mental stupor, the spider might not spin at all.

--Spiders on morphine took 3 hours to spin webs which they had previously spun in 20 minutes.

--Spiders on tranquilizers did not spin the longest, most complicated strands of their webs.

--Spiders on LSD were energetic, but spun useless "free form" webs.

--Spiders in one study spun rectangular rather than the normal circular webs, after exposure to marijuana.

If the photos below do not show on your reader—click:
http://www.trinity.edu/jdunn/spiderdrugs.htm

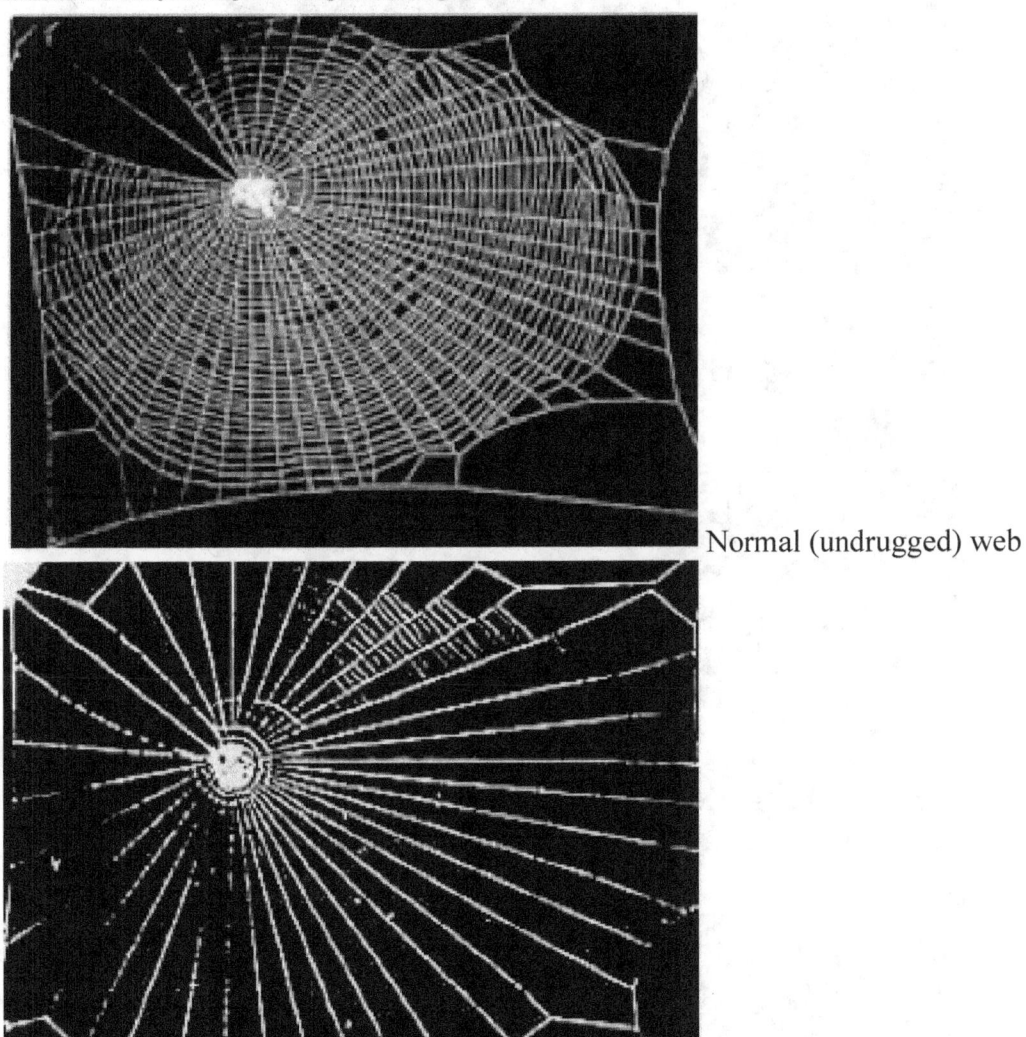

Normal (undrugged) web

Web spun under peyote/mescaline

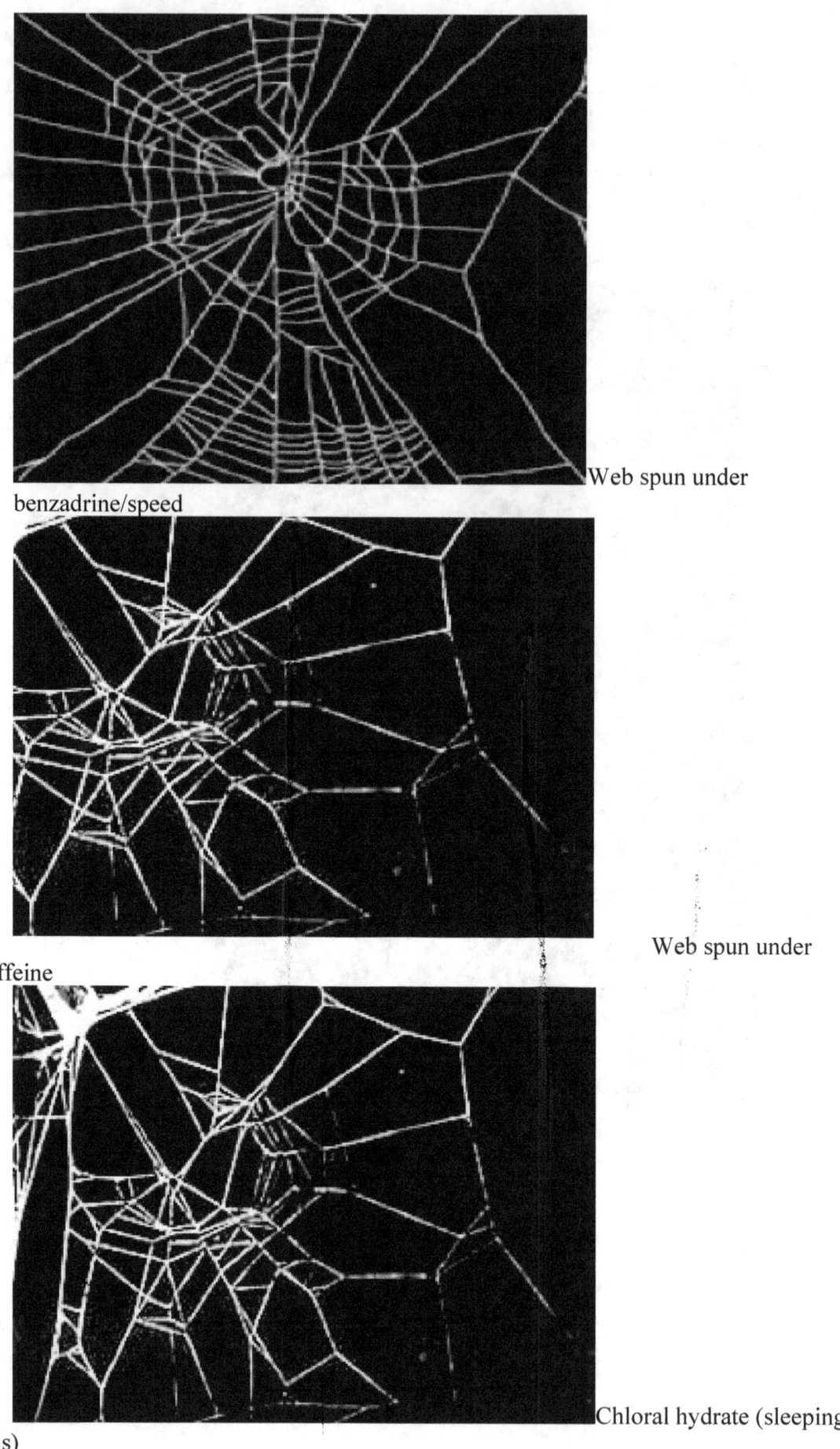

Web spun under benzadrine/speed

Web spun under Caffeine

Chloral hydrate (sleeping pills)

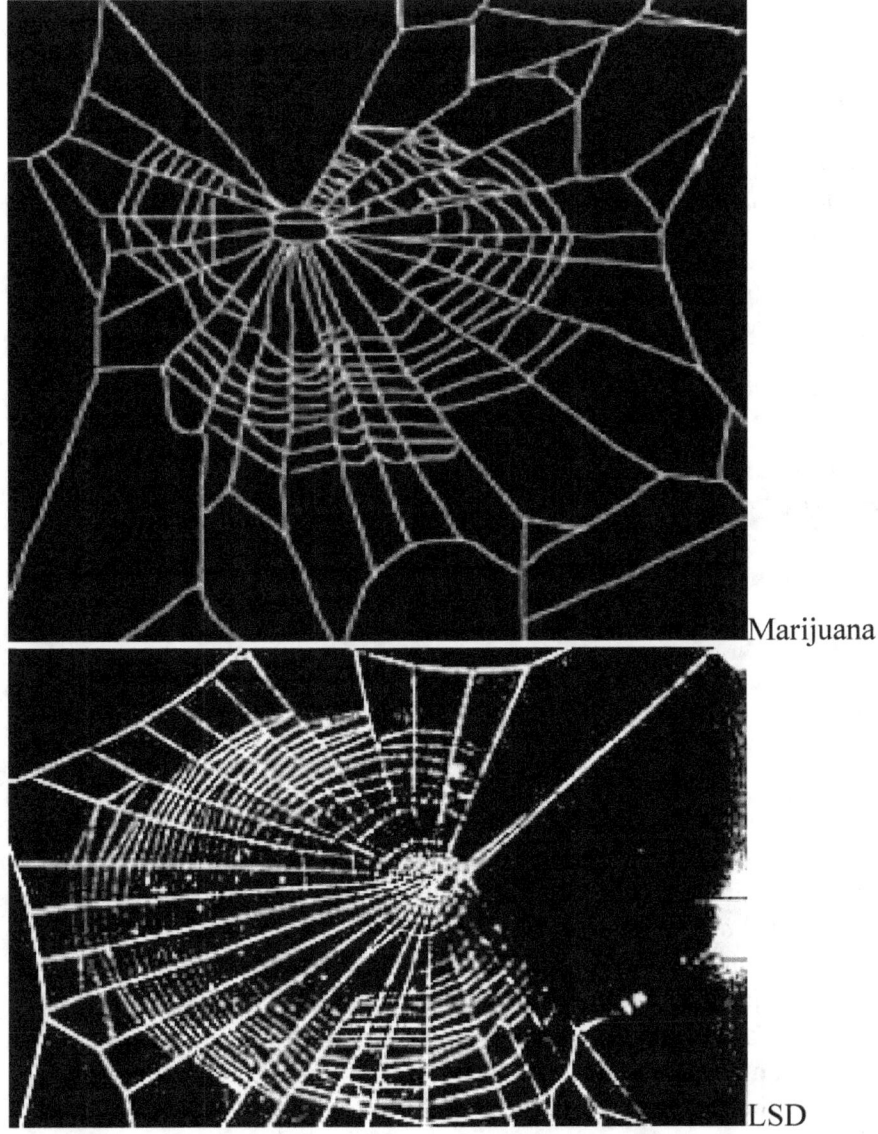

Marijuana

LSD

The use of psychoactive drugs is a symptom which should alert us to the deep underlying problems. No matter how much we hear people rationalize their drug use by saying that they want "pleasure now," We should be able to recognize that the overwhelming reasons for illegal and excessive drug use is a lack of need fulfillment, insecurity, inferiority complexes (frustrated power drive), lack of self-esteem, or a lack of love. These are the real reasons that push most people into retreating from reality through drugs.

The reasons that one might use dangerous or potentially dangerous drugs range from experimentation (curiosity), to being "one of the gang" (as a means of feeling secure or gaining the esteem of others), to relaxing, to retreating from reality occasionally, to the continual retreat from reality. Obviously the latter is the most severe. It is in this category that the users have developed uncontrollable needs for a drug--a mental dependence (habit) or a physical dependence of their bodies (addiction).

The people who use the mind altering drugs, and those who choose not to, are often separated by basic value choices. The drug user tends to see "pleasure now" as being more important than planning and working for the future. They also tend to be rather passive in their approaches to life. Withdrawing from the "rat race" is chosen over the goal of doing what is "right" and doing one's duty. They give up the possibility of accomplishing worthwhile goals, developing their self esteem, or becoming "truly human" as Maslow advocated.

Psychoactive drugs work by affecting the nerves or the synapses, the spaces between the nerves between the nerves. The electrical impulse moves down the nerve to its terminal, the end of the nerve. The dendrites, the tree-like branches at the terminal release a chemical, called a neurotransmitter. This chemical moves across the synaptic gap and stimulates the dendrites on the

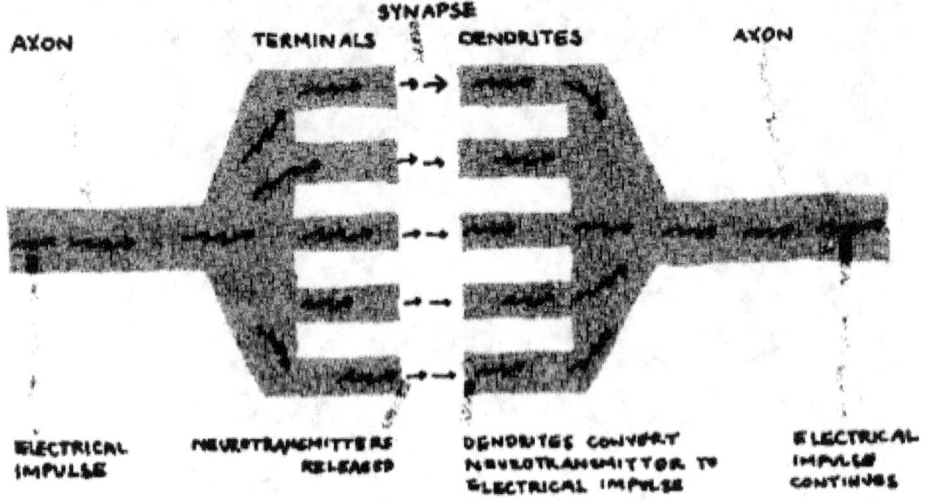

next
nerve. This starts a new electrical impulse which will travel down that nerve. This action of electrical impulse to neurotransmitter, to electrical impulse, to neurotransmitter may happen several hundred times as the nerve pathway delivers a message.

Drugs work in the synapse by:

---increasing the amount of neurotransmitter released;

---imitating the action of the neurotransmitter;

---slowing the reabsorption of the neurotransmitter whithatisch should return to the terminal so that it can be used again, this therefore increases the amount of neurotransmitter in the synapse;

--- slowing the release of the neurotransmitter.

Alcohol works on the nerve fibers, slowing down or stopping that fiber from carrying the electrical impulse. It also works, as do other drugs, in the synapses and increases or decreases the effect of the neurotransmitters.

Over 200 neurotransmitters have been found. For the purposes of this book we will mention only four of the most common: norepinephrine, dopamine (both have stimulating effects), and acetylcholine and serotonin (which have calming effects). We had earlier mentioned GABA as a neurotransmitter which can affect the experience of a drug user, but from this point on we will mention only the other four major neurotransmitters. These neurotransmitters are necessary to everyday functioning. A lack or an excess of one or more of them can cause mental problems. For example: Too much dopamine in one area of the brain has been associated with schizophrenia. Not enough dopamine in another area has been associated with depression. A lack of serotonin makes it difficult to relax and to sleep. An insufficient amount of norepinephrine or serotonin in some areas of the brain can make us forget--and may be associated with Alzheimer's disease. There is also a great deal of research to show that both suicide and aggressive behavior are related to the levels of serotonin, dopamine, and norepinephrine related compounds.

When the neurotransmitters are used and depleted by the action of drugs, or the effects of aging, the person's mood and energy level will be affected. Since neurotransmitters are made from amino acids sometimes a diet rich in the amino acids can help to rebuild them. The amino acid choline is used to make acetylcholine. Phenylalanine is used to make dopamine. And, norepinephrine is made from dopamine.

There may be help for aging people whose neurotransmitters have been reduced. In early experiments by Timothy Collier at the University of Rochester, senile rats who had lost their memories were given implants of the norepinephrine producing cells from young rats. They regained memory. In another experiment he implanted cells which make needed nerve growth factor (NGF) into rats whose nerve cells had died. With the new NGF the dead nerve cells began to regenerate.

THE PLEASURE PATHWAYS OR THE PLEASURE CENTER OF THE BRAIN

As an example of how a drug may affect a person, you might imagine a person using a drug that affects the hypothalamus. This organ monitors both body temperature and hunger. A drug which changes the neurotransmitter output here might make the person feel more hungry or feel full. If the drug affected the temperature mechanism it might make the person feel hot or cold.

Some people using PCP ("angel dust") felt very hot because of the action on the hypothalamus from that drug. It was not uncommon to have a person who was under the influence of PCP take off all of his or her clothes because of feeling very hot. At the beach when a person felt hot because of PCP there was all that water in which to cool off. One problem was that even if the person was a good swimmer, it is common to forget how to swim. Consequently there were a number of drownings due to PCP ingestion.

Cocaine and its derivatives, as well as the amphetamines, stimulate the neurotransmitters in the pleasure center (medial forebrain bundle) at the end of the hypothalamus. During sexual intercourse it is this area which is excited and gives the pleasure of an orgasm. Cocaine can give a similar, often more intense, orgasmic feeling.

The release of dopamine and serotonin in the nucleus accumbens lies at the root of active drug addiction. The pattern of neural firing that results from this surge of neurotransmitters is the "high." It is the chemical essence of what it means to be addicted. Part of the medial forebrain bundle (MFB), which mediates punishment and reward, the nucleus accumbens, is the ultimate target for the dopamine released by the ingestion of cocaine, for example.

The release of dopamine and serotonin in the nucleus accumbens appears to be the final destination of the reward pathway. If you think about a drug, take a drug, or crave a drug, brain scans will show that you are stimulating the nucleus accumbens with a surge of electrochemical activity. This in shown as an increase in color on the scan. The same reward pathways have been identified as essentially the same as those that regulate our food and water-seeking behavior. By directly or indirectly influencing the molecules of pleasure, drugs and alcohol trigger key neurochemical events that are central to our feelings of both reward and disappointment. In this sense, the reward pathway is a route to both pleasure and pain.

Alcohol, heroin, cigarettes, and other drugs cause a surge of dopamine production, which is then released into the nucleus accumbens. The result is pleasure—or at least a reduction in pain. When scientists inject a dopamine-mimicking substance into the nucleus accumbens, targeting dopamine receptors, withdrawal symptoms are blocked in morphine-addicted rats. Similarly, when scientists block dopamine receptors in the accumbens, the morphine-dependent rats exhibit withdrawal symptoms.

When one removes large slices of the nucleus accumbens, animals no longer want the drugs. So, one cure for addiction has been discovered already—but surgically removing chunks of the midbrain of people just won't do, of course.

Dopamine is more than a primary pleasure chemical—a "happy hormone," as it has been called. Dopamine is also the key molecule involved in the memory of pleasurable acts. Dopamine is part of the reason why a person remembers how much he liked getting high yesterday.

The fact that we know all this is nothing short of amazing, but it is part of a larger perspective afforded by the insights of contemporary neurobiology. We know, for example, that the emotion of fear arises, in large part, through chemical changes in a peanut-sized limbic organ called the amygdala. Does this information make fear any less fearful? It merely locates the brain area upon which the sensation of fear is built.

Craving has a biological basis. Studies of the nucleus accumbens have demonstrated abnormal firing rates in scanned addicts who were deep into an episode of craving. The craving for a reward that is not forthcoming causes dopamine levels in the nucleus accumbens to crash dramatically, as they do when users go off drugs. On the other hand, dopamine, serotonin, and norepinephrine activity soars dramatically when a drug user relieves withdrawal symptoms by relapsing. So drug hunger in abstinent addicts is not all in the head, or strictly psychological.

THE NERVOUS SYSTEM AND THE EFFECTS OF DRUGS

The cerebral cortex is the outside part of the brain. The frontal area is more involved in thinking. The sides are the sites of feelings and movement of the body. Hearing is done in a lower area on the side. Vision is registered at the back of the brain. Many drugs affect this area. Alcohol can deaden any area. Stimulants can excite any area. Hallucinogenics may alter the impulses, particularly in the vision and hearing areas.

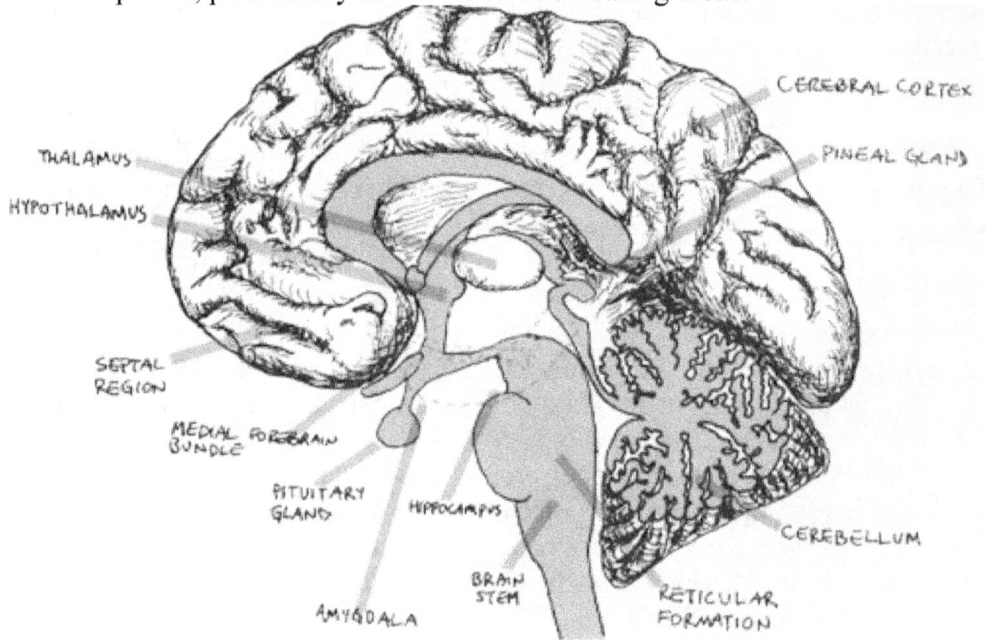

The reticular activating system, or reticular formation, is located at the base of the brain on the top of the brain stem. All impulses which come from the body to the brain or from the brain to the body go through this area. This area controls the "arousal" state of the brain and determines our alertness to information being transmitted. A drug which affects the reticular activating system (such as alcohol) can modify the messages being sent in either direction.

The hypothalamus is a major control center for the body. Among its functions are the previously mentioned monitoring of hunger and body temperature.

The medial forebrain bundle (pleasure center) is a bundle of nerves in the front part of the hypothalamus. The pleasure of orgasm is a function of this area. Cocaine and amphetamines are major stimulators of this area but opium derivatives and marijuana also can slightly modify this area.

The periventricular system is also known as the "discomfort center." This has an opposite effect from the pleasure center. No one would voluntarily take a drug to stimulate this area and make them feel bad.

Because the blood flow to the brain is greater than in any other organ every substance in the blood is found in greater amounts in the brain. Whether it is vitamin C (which has no affect on the brain), aspirin, alcohol, or cocaine--the brain will be more affected than any other organ.

108

The Most Commonly Abused Drugs may be classified as depressants, stimulants, cannabis, and hallucinogenics.

Depressants

The depressants are those drugs that slow the activity of the brain or body. They slow the beating of the heart, take blood away from the surface of the body, slow the breathing rate, and slow the reactions. They may be used to induce sleep, to relax, to kill pain and to control certain abnormal brain activity such as is found in epilepsy. The most commonly abused depressants are: alcohol, barbiturates, tranquilizers, narcotics, and inhalants or solvents.

The depressants or "downers" are apt to develop physical dependence in the abuser of the drug. There is also a great deal of danger to infants born to depressant-abusing mothers. Newborn infants undergoing withdrawal from the drug taken by the mother is not uncommon. This can happen to babies whose mothers are alcoholics, opiate users, or abusers of any of the other downers which cause physical dependence.

All "downers" depress the brain and its functions to some degree. Since there are parts of the brain which inhibit certain actions, these inhibiting areas can also be depressed. That is why a person using a depressant may act excited. If a person has been inhibiting hostile feelings, a depressant may make that person want to argue or fight. If a person has been shy, the effects of the depressant may make that person feel more socially confident. Other people just want to relax or sleep when under the influence of a downer. So the effect of the depressant depends on the type of drug, the dosage and the personality of the user.

Barbiturates are central nervous system depressants which are used as sleeping pills and sedatives. They derive their name from the chemical, barbituric acid, which is their major ingredient. The milder barbiturates are called sedatives that is, they calm and relax the user. In stronger forms or higher doses they are hypnotic, or sleep producing.

The dangers of barbiturate use include the possibilities of psychic dependence, physical dependence, and death. There is a great likelihood of physical addiction to these drugs. And the withdrawal from them is more severe than is withdrawal from heroin. Barbiturate withdrawal may lead to death; heroin withdrawal is almost never a cause of death. Because of the dangers inherent in barbiturate withdrawal it should be done under the care of a physician.

Death due to barbiturate poisoning far exceeds the deaths from heroin. And there are more barbiturate deaths than there are deaths from all other drugs combined. There may be several reasons for the high death rate attributed to this class of drugs. One is that while the user develops a tolerance for the drug, needing more to get a lesser effect, the lethal dose does not increase proportionately as it does with the opiates. A second reason is that barbiturate sleeping pills are usually easily obtained through prescription or from illegal sales. They are therefore quite handy for intentional overdose by those who are suicidal. A third reason for the high death rate is that barbiturates when taken with alcohol multiply the effects of each. So a few drinks and a few barbiturate sleeping pills can result in accidental death.

TRANQUILLIZERS

The tranquilizers are "daytime depressants." Their stated purpose is to relieve mental tension and anxieties and, in some cases, to relax the muscles. These drugs are also used to prevent motion sickness. They should not cause one to sleep. However, many of them may induce sleep, especially in larger than normal doses. The minor tranquilizers are generally prescribed for people who are outside of mental hospitals and who need some chemical help to control their tensions. These generally work by reducing the neurotransmitters in the sympathetic nervous system--particularly norepinephrine, while also reducing the parasympathetic neurotransmitters which allow one to sleep--particularly serotonin. So they should theoretically act by reducing tensions while keeping one awake.

109

The minor tranquilizers are much less toxic than the barbiturates, but still carry the disadvantage of depressed mental alertness. Therefore, people in hazardous occupations or people who must drive an automobile should be aware that their alertness is decreased.

Tolerance develops slowly to tranquilizers, but physical dependence is highly possible. These drugs also develop a cross tolerance with alcohol and barbiturates so that being tolerant to one creates a tolerance to the others.

NARCOTICS

The narcotics are either derived from the opium poppy (codeine, heroin, morphine) or are synthetically made so that they are chemically similar to the natural opium products (demerol, methadone, Darvon, Meperidine). The narcotics numb the senses which relieves pain and produces sleepiness. They may be used by physicians for these purposes. Opium derivatives are used in paregoric (opium and camphor) to control diarrhea and in cough medicines (as codeine) to suppress the cough impulse. While the narcotics may vary in strength, from the mild form of codeine to the very strong heroin, they are all dangerous because of their potential for addiction.

Opium is little used in America because it is too bulky to transport into the country. When it is used it is usually smoked or swallowed. During the 18th and 19th centuries several remedies containing opium were developed in America and England. By the late 1800's about one American in 400 was addicted to opium. In the 1700's the Chinese attempted to make opium use illegal because the addiction was severely hurting the country. But the British, who were selling Indian opium to the Chinese, fought a war (the Opium War of 1839-1842) to insure that the Chinese would continue to buy and use their opium. Things really haven't changed much have they? Somebody is always trying to make a buck on us!

Codeine is made from morphine. It is not as strong as morphine nor is it as addictive. Today it is used in many cough suppressants and is often combined with aspirin or Tylenol to make a more potent pain killer.

Withdrawal from any of the opiates is marked by a hyper-excitability, shaking, cramps, sweating, chills, nausea, etc.

THE STIMULANTS

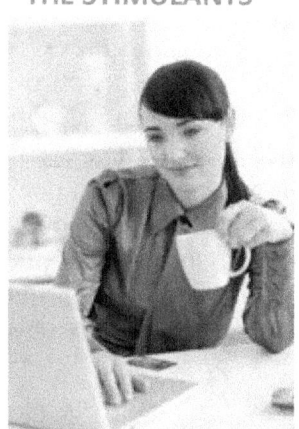

Stimulants are those drugs that "pep up" or stimulate the central nervous system. They speed up the neural firing so that the nerve cells act as super transmitters. People using stimulants, then, use their energy resources at faster than normal speeds. They may decrease fatigue, increase alertness, and make the user more energetic for a time. However, after a while there is a great increase in the amount of fatigue and the user becomes more irritable and may develop headaches.

Caffeine is found in coffee, tea and cola drinks as well as in some pills designed to keep the user awake. It is the leading mind altering drug in use in America. One of the effects of caffeine is the increasing of the firing rates of the neurons, which makes the person feel more alert. This may increase a person's ability to learn, at least it has been shown to help rats to learn. The alertness which the caffeine in two to four cups of coffee develops can also assist in improving drivers' reaction time. However, caffeine pills are not a substitute for the coffee. They tend to make the users nervous and irritable.

Other research has indicated that the stimulating effects of the caffeine may be a factor in heart disease. In a study of 12, 000 patients by the Boston Inter-hospital Group it was concluded that coffee (including decaffeinated coffee) is a causative agent in heart disease. Other studies do not necessarily confirm this finding. Depending on the study, caffeine has been found to be a risk factor in heart disease and not a risk factor.

Coffee is a more potent stimulant than is generally recognized. It contains about 90 milligrams of caffeine per six ounce cup. Decaffeinated coffee contains about 1 milligram per cup. And tea contains about 45 milligrams per cup. The therapeutic dose for people overdosed on barbiturates is 43 milligrams, less than half that in a cup of coffee.

ENERGY DRINKS

In 1997 the "energy drink" Red Bull became initially available in the United States. It was first introduced to Austria in 1987. Since then many more "energy drinks" have become available and there has been a lot of research on the harmful effects of their use. There is no FDA regulation and the United States has no bans. However, in other countries the use and marketing of "energy drinks" is banned.

Along with caffeine many of the "Energy Drinks" include other ingredients such as; taurine, glucoronolactone, guarana, B vitamins, and hormonal additives. With all of this there is much documented evidence of harmful side effects and high risk health behaviors such as; increased aggression, sexual risk taking, increased substance use, and even failure to use safety devices such as seat belts and motorcycle or bicycle helmets. The common occurrence of using "Energy Drinks" along with alcohol can add to these detrimental effects. (6)

COCAINE

Cocaine Lcocaine hydrochloride) is the most potent "natural" stimulant. Some of the "street names" are "coke," "snow," or "blow." It is made from the leaves of the coca bush which grows in Java and parts of South America. Cocaine has an anesthetic effect if applied to the skin, but is a stimulant if taken internally. The drug is usually sniffed ("snorted") with its effects beginning in 5 to 15 minutes, but can be injected for a high which begins almost immediately.

Several neurotransmitters, but particularly dopamine, are involved. Like many other drugs which are now abused, cocaine was once used medically. Sigmund Freud prescribed it as a substitute for aspirin and as an aid to withdrawal from morphine. But he soon learned of its ill effects when many of the people of Vienna became psychologically dependent on the drug.

Tolerance to cocaine develops quickly. More is needed as the neurotransmitters in the synapses are exhausted by the high output caused by the cocaine. Scientists have detected a 50% drop in dopamine in only ten days in rats who had been given cocaine.11 After the "high" a fairly rapid depression may set in, so the user again needs the cocaine to bring back the pleasant effects of the drug. Long term use of the drug does not increase one's tolerance to the lethal dose, in fact in some cases, because of the weakened condition of the body, the lethal dose may be much less than would be expected.

Some people mix cocaine with heroin to prolong the "high." They call this mixture a "speedball." This combination can lead to the expected psychological and physical dependence on cocaine as well as a physical addiction to the heroin. Several celebrities (such as John Belushi and River Phoenix) have died because of the effects of speedballs.

Free base cocaine is a much purer form of the drug. It can be over 98% pure. After the non-active ingredients are removed the cocaine "base" is left. It is usually smoked. The high, of course, is exceptionally quick and strong.

Crack cocaine is a solid form of cocaine made from dissolving the cocaine hydrochloride with an alkaline substance such as baking soda. The small "rocks" of cocaine that are left are smoked. It, too, gives an intense high. It is also far more addicting than normal cocaine. It is this crack which is the common drug of the ghettos--and the basis of a drug trade which has been exported around the country by ghetto gangs such as the Crips and the Bloods.

Among the problems of cocaine and its derivatives are: heart attacks and strokes (due to the extreme excitement to the central nervous system and the major body organs), a stoppage of breathing (due to a cramping of the diaphragm (the major breathing muscle), a feeling that there are bugs under the skin (vermification) which is caused by the hyper-excitability of the nerves, and when the drug is "snorted" a breakdown of the nasal septum (the cartilage that divides the nostrils) which is caused by the intense constriction then dilation of the blood vessels in the nose. As little as 20 milligrams is enough to kill some sensitive people but the average lethal dose is 1200 milligrams.

Cocaine also is a major factor in birth defects and "the use of cocaine among pregnant mothers is skyrocketing". Cocaine not only crosses the placenta of a pregnant mother but it is actually carried on the sperm. It then causes damage to nerves and blood vessels. Cocaine use by the mother during pregnancy is also related to an increase in the Sudden Infant Death Syndrome in babies.(2)

AMPHETAMINES

The amphetamines are very potent stimulants. They are synthetically made to stimulate the secretion of adrenaline or to mimic the action of adrenaline. They are, therefore, stimulants of the central nervous system. Medically they are used to: keep people awake if they have an uncontrollable impulse to sleep (narcolepsy); to control some children who are overactive (hyperkinetic); or to suppress hunger in people wishing to lose weight. But all three of these behavior problems may be related to psychological problems rather than physical problems. For that reason, especially in the area of weight reducing, amphetamines are not necessarily the answer to the problem.

Among the negative effects of amphetamine abuse are: high blood pressure, delusions, psychotic reactions, permanent brain damage, and death. Babies of amphetamine abusing mothers have been born with deformed hearts. Although the drugs are often taken by students to get them started with homework, they do not improve performance, and may increase errors. While many people take the drugs to gain energy, the energy they feel does not come from the drug, but rather from the food that they have consumed. But since the amphetamines speed up the use of calories while suppressing the appetite amphetamine users may lose excessive amounts of weight. This often requires hospitalization.

Methamphetamine (Crank, speed, ice, meth) is the most powerful form of amphetamines. It can be smoked, injected, snorted, or taken in pill form. In the past heavy stimulant drug users chose whichever drug was cheapest at the time--cocaine or amphetamines. Today with both becoming cheaper both are used.

In the 1960's hippies who used "speed" found that death often accompanied their highs. Consequently the saying "Speed kills" became popular--and most of the 60's drug users avoided methamphetamines. Today, unaware of the experience of the earlier drug culture of the hippies, many people are using cocaine, crack cocaine, methamphetamines, or a combination of crack and speed called "croak."

The dependence on amphetamines leads to withdrawal symptoms which include severe depression, hallucinations, and paranoid suspicions. It is therefore important that a doctor supervise withdrawal from these "uppers". They are considered so dangerous that Sweden totally outlawed them years ago. Many countries have since followed suit.

Synthetic upper drugs which mimic amphetamines or cocaine, but are usually much stronger than cocaine, have hit the market. "Cat" (methcathinone) is one such powerful drug. These drugs are extremely dangerous often leading to paranoia, severe weight loss, and suicidal thoughts.

MDMA (3-4-methylenedioxymethamphetamine) or Ecstasy , is a synthetic drug with amphetamine-like and hallucinogenic properties. Because of its stimulant qualities it is often taken at "raves" and parties where endurance-dancing is expected. It generally increases one's feeling of self-confidence. It often also makes the user feel closer to others and often increases one's desire to touch other people. It increases the heart rate and blood pressure and has been known to cause death. As with other uppers, withdrawing can cause sleep problems, anxiety and depression. Long-term use may damage the cells that produce serotonin, so one's mood, appetite, learning and memory may be negatively affected.

CANNABIS

Cannabis is the term internationally used to indicate the family of hallucinogenic containing hemp plants (cannabis sativa). These hemp plants are often used to make rope. Although America does not cultivate the plants for this reason, preferring to import Manila hemp or synthetic fibers such as nylon.

The flowering tops of the plants, especially the female plant, hold a resin which contains an hallucinogenic compound called Delta 9-THC (tetrahydrocannabinol). After the plants (leaves, seed, flowers, stems) are dried they may be smoked or eaten in order to achieve the desired effects. Users have reported various effects from the drug--stimulant, depressant, or hallucinogenic. It is smoked by about 22 million people in the United States--6 million smoke it daily. However the use is reducing yearly.

THC is a very strong hallucinogenic, one of several psychoactive chemicals in marijuana. But the dosage and the method of ingestion give it varying effects. The marijuana grown the United States has usually ranged from 0 to 4% but can go over 20%. The average joint is becoming stronger. In the 1970s the THC in a marijuana joint averaged about 1%. Twenty years later it was closer to 4%. Some strains of marijuana can have a THC level over 25%. The Federal Government is raising marijuana with THC percentages of 2 to 4%. This is to be used for government experiments relating to the effects of marijuana.

As you might conclude, if you are researching marijuana and don't know what level of THC is in the marijuana that you are working with, your studies are not likely to be valid or reliable. It would be like a person studying alcohol and comparing light beer with 150 proof rum. This is a problem when studying marijuana or when comparing marijuana to alcohol.

There are two major species of cannabis, cannabis sativa and cannabis induca. Cannabis sativa is the taller variety and its effects tend to be linked to feelings of relaxation, giddiness and hunger. Cannabis indica has a more conical shape with broader leaves. It is more likely to give a more stoned, some say, "meditative' feeling. Some believe that it is because of a higher cannibidiol to THC ratio. Cannibidiol does not have much of a psychoactive effect but it is believed that it may act to increase the effect of THC.(3) A minor species, at least in terms of its psychoactive use, is cannabis ruderalis which grows wild in much of central Asia.

THC raises the pulse rate and blood pressure of marijuana smokers. Its effect on the body is stronger than the nicotine in cigarettes. In many parts of the world psychotic reactions to THC are relatively common, especially to first time users. In America, because of the low dosage of the weed, such reactions are very rare.

THC, or its chemical by-products, have a half-life of 7 to 10 days, although various studies have placed it between 1 1/2 days to three weeks. Habitual users show longer half-lives. A half-life means that half of the THC will be gone in about a week, half of the remainder in another week, and so forth. It takes about 4 1/2 months after one has stopped using marijuana or hashish to reduce the amount THC that was present at that time to 1%. This may account for the "reverse tolerance" which is often evidenced by marijuana users. They need less of the drug to get the same high.

The longer half-life is due in part to the fact that THC is fat soluble. Alcohol, on the other hand, is water soluble so has a shorter half-life--usually less than a day. This long half-life of THC is responsible for the fact that marijuana damage is called duration-related, while alcohol damage is called dose-related. This means that alcohol damage depends on the amount of alcohol consumed in a single bout. But marijuana damage is more related to how long the drug has been used rather than how much was used at one time.

Marijuana (dope, pot, grass) is the dried parts of the cannabis plant. It may be put into food (like brownies) or made into a solution (like tea), but it is usually smoked. It does not look or smell like tobacco, being green in color and alfalfa-like in smell.

The psychological effects of marijuana may be somewhat influenced by what the user expects. In Jamaica it may be used as a stimulant to allow people to work faster in the sugar cane fields. Conversely, in the United States people usually use it to relax. Here they may get hungry while using it ("the munchies") but in Portugal the fishermen often use it to avoid hunger while on their daily fishing trips.

In the early 1980's the average joint of marijuana contained about 1/2 of 1% THC. It

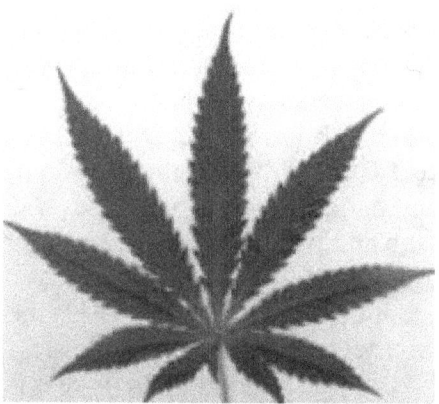

was very weak. Today it can range from 1/2 to 12% THC--stronger than the hashish of a few years ago. Varieties of the weed from Vietnam, Thailand, and Jamaica are quite high in THC. But the highest THC ratio is found in Sinsemilla--a hybrid female plant.

The psychological effects of marijuana on the user vary depending on the dose of the drug, the personality of the user, and what the user expects to happen. For example, in one study done at U. C. L. A., people who expected to get "high" were given marijuana containing no THC. They got "high". Others, who thought that nothing would happen to them if they smoked the drug were given marijuana with 3% THC--and they generally felt no effects.

Does marijuana cause brain damage? A British study of ten chronic marijuana smokers found evidence of brain atrophy. A study at Tulane University found microscopic evidence of damage done to monkeys who had been forced to smoke marijuana. A study conducted at the University of Pennsylvania Medical School implied that there seemed to be some change in the brains of chronic marijuana smokers. A number of studies have indicated the possibility of damage to smoking marijuana. They may be true, but there are a number of problems with the studies. For example early studies on monkeys who were forced to smoke a great deal of marijuana showed brain damage. But the amount of marijuana smoke was far more than would be expected in normal human smokers. Another problem is that marijuana smokers may also smoke cigarettes, drink alcohol or use other psychoactive drugs so it is very difficult to isolate the effects of marijuana alone. It is also difficult to determine the amount of THC in the joints smoked. Of course it may not be the THC but some of the 400 other ingredients in the smoke that do damage. Then would there be a damage difference among those who smoked through water pipes compared to those who did not. And what about those who ate marijuana-laced brownies? Then there are the variables in measuring the damage. Should be done in autopsies, by brain scans or by verbal and written testing to indicate any effects to brain function. In

114

addition we might want to know the condition of the brain of the user before he or she has never smoked marijuana. So while there are studies concluding that there is brain damage and that there is not brain damage, there are so many variables that it is difficult to determine with any degree of certainty. But then brain damage is actually a relatively small element in the psychological and social effects of marijuana use. Recent evidence (4) indicates that there are other problems related to marijuana use. A study at the University of Iowa testing various mental abilities and physical coordinations for marijuana smokers and a placebo group that held its breath for both short and long periods of time found that marijuana smokers, compared to placebo smokers, had most of their mental skills reduced. The exceptions were in vocabulary and abstract thinking. Their manipulative skills, which might be important in driving a car, were impaired. The placebo smokers had four of their mental skills reduced just from breath holding.

There is of course the possible link to cancer. Distillate of marijuana smoke and of cigarette smoke can cause cancer on mouse skins and the amount of benzopyrene, unknown cancer producer, is 70% higher in marijuana smoke than in tobacco smoke. Other studies have shown reduced immune system reaction due to some effects of marijuana smoke. This is the same effect found in tobacco smoke. While some pro-marijuana advocates have suggested smoking through a water pipe, the tars are not water soluble so they still enter the lungs and the water has only a small effect on the amount of carbon monoxide inhaled. What the water does is to reduce the damage to the mucous membranes from the heat of the smoke.

But it is the mental effects of marijuana that concern most people. Dr. Louis West of UCLA, a long time marijuana researcher, found out after observing marijuana users for three years, that some of them had personality changes. He also found apathy, an inability to concentrate, an impaired skill in communicating with others, a loss of insight, and fragmentation in the flow of their thoughts. Studies in the Netherlands have indicated a strong correlation between the heaviness of smoking marijuana and a schizophrenic's chances of relapse into the disease after receiving medical treatment. Heavy users (more than one joint daily) relapsed 61% of the time, light users relapsed 18% of the time, and non-users relapsed less than 6% of the time. The researchers were not certain whether the marijuana interfered with the medicine they were given or that marijuana users are more vulnerable to stressful life events which can cause a relapse.

DRUG DEPENDENCE

Psychological dependence is the term used when the mind believes that it needs a substance. The term habituated (having developed the habit) to the drug or other substance was an earlier term used to indicate this psychological dependence. While a person may become dependent on having chocolate ice cream or any other substance every day, what we really mean by drug dependence is the continued need for a mood altering drug. That drug may be caffeine, nicotine, alcohol, heroin, or any other upper, downer, or hallucinogenic .

Many people have become accustomed to the stimulating effect of caffeine, so they drink several cups of coffee or several glasses of cola each day. Some people have become dependent on the stimulant or the relaxant effect of cigarettes, so they smoke a pack or two daily. Many people feel the need for tranquilizers each day to relax or barbiturates each evening to sleep. These are common forms of drug dependence.

Physical dependence or addiction occurs when the body develops a physical need for the drug. The World Health Organization now prefers the term "physical dependence" to the commonly used term "addiction". This physical dependence on the drug occurs with both "uppers" (cocaine, amphetamines, nicotine, caffeine) and "downers' (such as barbiturates, tranquilizers, alcohol and nicotine). The withdrawal symptoms from cocaine are obviously much stronger than from caffeine. And the withdrawal from nicotine is often quite noticeable because one is withdrawing from both an upper effect and a downer effect.

The downers or depressants depress the central nervous system. They depress the output of nervous energy by the body. But the body attempts to stay normal (homeostasis) so it puts out more energy. Because the body is putting out more energy, the drug user must use more of the depressant to overcome the energy of the body.

When the person who is physically dependent stops taking the depressant drug, the excess energy being developed over-stimulates the body. The excess of nervous impulses causes cramps in the muscles, nausea, chills, sweating, and other painful effects. These are known as withdrawal symptoms. and feel depressed. The initial crash can take from a few hours to four days. During this time there is intense depression, anxiety, agitation, and a craving for the drug. For the next one to ten weeks there is more anxiety and continued craving.

Years ago people thought that one could not be addicted to cocaine because a person coming off of cocaine did not have the withdrawal symptoms associated with heroin. Now it is realized that withdrawing from uppers and downers develop quite opposite effects on the body. A downer drug merely develops hyper-excitability, such as muscle cramps, while an upper drug withdrawal is a painfully depressing set of symptoms. And these withdrawals from uppers may be far more painful than the withdrawing from the downer drugs.

Tolerance to many drugs develops with excessive use. When increased doses are required to achieve the desired effect it is a sign that one has developed a tolerance to that drug. This can happen with medications such as antibiotics, where the disease causing organisms build up a certain immunity to the medicine so that more of the drug is required to control the infection. And it is common with the use of many mood altering drugs.

Drug dependent people who use "downers" (such as barbiturates, opiates and alcohol) often develop a tolerance for the drugs. They need to increase the doses continually in order to get the same effect that was once achieved in a small dose. A normal dose of morphine to control pain would be 10 to 20 milligrams. The lethal dose of the drug is assumed to be about 200 milligrams. But morphine addicts have been known use as much as 5,000 milligrams--25 times the dose that should be fatal. Barbiturates, on the other hand, have a normal therapeutic dose of 100 to 200 milligrams, but tolerance to the sedative effects of the drug develops so that the user may need to increase the dosage. But the fatal dosage of 1,000 to 2,000 milligrams is not significantly raised as the user increases the dosage. It is, therefore, much easier to overdose with barbiturates than with the opiates such as morphine or heroin.

Tolerance to some drugs occurs because the liver makes extra enzymes with which to break down the drugs. With more enzymes available the drug is broken down faster so more of the drug is needed to get the same effect as a lower dose once gave. Similarly, with alcohol tolerance the increased enzymes metabolize the alcohol faster.

Cross tolerance occurs when one drug increases the body's tolerance to itself and to one or more other drugs. Alcohol, valium, and barbiturates are cross tolerant. If you are tolerant to alcohol then give up the alcohol for Valium or barbiturates, you will be tolerant to the other drug also. You will notice that not all "downer" drugs are cross tolerant. The opiates are not among those drugs that develop the same body tolerance as the other downers. However, the several types of opiates develop a cross tolerance to each other. In another family of drugs, the hallucinogens, such as LSD, psilocybin, and mescaline-- is a huge also develop a tolerance for each other.

Reverse tolerance occurs when a person needs less of a drug to get the same effect. As alcohol destroys the liver there is less liver to metabolize it so a lesser amount of alcohol can have a longer intoxicating effect. So it is possible, with alcohol, to have a tolerance and a reverse tolerance at the same time--as the enzymes per ounce of liver increase but the weight of the liver tissue decreases.

Fat soluble drugs, such as marijuana (THC) and PCP remain in the body for long periods of time. Since it is already in the body, it is therefore possible to get a desired effect without taking in as much of the drug.

ADDICTION (SUBSTANCE DEPENDANCE)

Over the years the word "addiction" has been defined, redefined and eliminated from our drug lexicon. The Diagnostic and Statistical Manual of Mental Disorders (DSM-IV) does not currently use the term, preferring "substance dependence" as the term of choice. Through the years it has been quite common to split the idea of substance dependence between that which was merely a habit (habituation) and that which was a physical reaction when the drug was not available.

So with alcohol a person might have a very strong desire to drink every night after work (habituation) or the person might have a physical withdrawal when alcohol was unavailable. This was called the DTs, delirium tremens. With heroin, there could be the strong desire to inject (habituation) or there could be the physical withdrawal symptoms of shaking and pain. This we had called addiction or physical dependence. So a person can have a very strong psychological desire for the physical and mental effects of a drug but not have physical withdrawal symptoms if the drug is not used.

When a person has a strong mental attachment to a substance it requires special types of therapies, which may or may not include the use of prescription medications. When one has the physical dependence medical assistance is either required or advisable so that if medications are needed they can be administered. Medication often reduces the pain that is part of the physical reaction to the loss of the drug.

The withdrawal of the drug such as caffeine or nicotine can usually be handled by oneself. Cocaine or amphetamine withdrawal are much more difficult. And withdrawal from barbiturates can be life-threatening.

TREATMENT

Treatment for drug abusers takes three major approaches. They may be given drugs. They may be separated from society. Or they may be treated psychologically. None have been greatly effective, so society often uses the least expensive means to alleviate the problem.

Often a physically dependent person must be isolated, either in a hospital where prescribed drugs can aid the withdrawal, or in a jail, where the withdrawal is often done "cold turkey" (without the aid of drugs). If in a hospital setting, the body must first be detoxified--the drug and its by-products must be removed from the body. Sometimes this takes several days or more. Often the physically dependent person can be aided in withdrawing from the addicting drugs and the withdrawal symptoms can be minimized by other medications.

The next step may be confinement in a jail, hospital or other treatment center. Sometimes convicted drug addicts are given a choice as to where they would like to be confined. And occasionally drug dependent people will voluntarily seek help through confinement. But confinement to a prison is not cheap for the taxpayers. The Department of Correction of California stated that it costs $30, 000 to build a jail cell, then $20,000 per year to keep a person in it. Methadone maintenance, on the other hand, costs about $2,000 per year.

Most people who honestly desire to rid themselves of their drug habits will commit themselves to a "Milieu treatment center." During a 2 to 6 week session the patient is first "detoxed." There is then a series of full day experiences including: therapy sessions, films, talks by former abusers, meetings with family members, Twelve Step Programs (such as those used by Alcoholics Anonymous), and other such experiences which assist the dependent person to become free from the need for drugs and to start an independent life.

The next step might be a "half-way house. " Communities of people who are or have been physically or mentally dependent on drugs have sprung up in many major cities. Phoenix House in New York is an example of these. In this type of institution the ex-addicts live together attempting to help each other to adjust to the real world from which they had withdrawn. Sometimes they work in the institution sponsored businesses, such as gas stations or shops. And usually there are encounter groups and other forms of psycho-therapy.

ALCOHOL

We are all familiar with the many reasons people give for their drinking. How many of these reasons are honest and how many are rationalizations? Have we evaluated the facts before making our decision on whether or how to use alcohol? What are the advantages and what are the disadvantages of alcohol use and what are the probabilities of our abusing the drug?

ALCOHOL--AMERICA'S MOST SERIOUS DRUG PROBLEM

Of all the methods used by people to withdraw from reality, alcohol is the most damaging to the American society. It damages people's brains and bodies, breaks up the stabilizing influence of the family, increases crime rates, costs businesses large amounts of money in lost time and in accidents, and it takes its toll on society in life, limb and money.

The National Commission of Marijuana and Drug Abuse has stated that "the use of alcohol (without question ... the most serious drug problem in the country today) and barbiturates (America's hidden drug problem) are condoned, but the use of marijuana and heroin are condemned." The commission deplored the inconsistency of these conflicting attitudes towards drugs, because alcohol is, indeed, a serious problem.

More than 85 million adults (79% of all adult males and 63% of all adult females) drink alcohol. One adult in 18 (4,800,000 total) is an alcoholic. An additional 5,000,000 are heavy drinkers, often called problem drinkers. Problem drinking, therefore, affects nearly one in every ten adults.

ALCOHOL THE CHEMICAL

Alcohol is formed when sugar in a plant is acted upon by yeast cells and thus broken down. The sugar in the plant yields both alcohol and carbon dioxide in this reaction. The action must take place without air. This is called fermentation. In some plants, notably grapes, apples and grains, the resulting alcohol can be consumed without death necessarily ensuing. This type of alcohol is called ethanol or ethyl alcohol. It is the intoxicating element in wine, beer, whisky, cough syrups and some "vitamin tonics." But it is also an inflammable solvent used in the manufacturing of chemicals, lacquers, explosives, gasoline additives, perfumes and in preserving specimens for laboratory use. The chemical formula for ethyl alcohol is $2\ C_2H_5OH$

Methyl alcohol is derived from the fermentation of wood products. There are some chemical similarities to ethanol, but if methyl alcohol is consumed it is a deadly poison which can cause blindness or death. Its chemical formula is CH_3OH.

Ethyl alcohol is soluble in water so is easily absorbed by the body. It is absorbed through the tongue and gums even before it is swallowed. Most of it is absorbed through the small intestine. And since alcohol requires no breakdown (digestion) it is absorbed rapidly after it is consumed.

The immediate effects on the body of ethyl alcohol include a speeding of the heart rate, a dilation of the blood vessels of the skin which makes one feel warmer. Alcohol is also a diuretic which causes the body to release fluids faster than usual. It does this by blocking the hormone which decreases urine flow. This causes excess urination which results in thirst a few hours later. There is also a decrease in sexual abilities. Shakespeare recognized this when he wrote that alcohol ". . . provokes the desire, but takes away from the performance." Most of us have also noted in others that when a person drinks there is a lack of attention span and a drop in muscular coordination.

The immediate effects of alcohol on the brain are substantial. Brain cells are destroyed even in normal social drinking. Heavy drinking has been estimated to destroy as many as 10,000 brain cells per drinking session. This brain cell destruction occurs because alcohol has a blood sludging effect on the red blood cells. They clump together and thereby slow down the blood flow. This, in turn, slows or stops the oxygen from entering the cells that need it. When this occurs in the brain, some cells die.

Blood sludging can also rupture small capillaries (blood vessels) and cause small hemorrhages. (This phenomenon also occurs in about 50 different diseases, including malaria and typhoid fever.) The sludging effect of alcohol can be observed in a person's eye capillaries after having consumed just one glass of beer.

Long term effects of drinking alcohol include: a propensity to a number of cancers, beer drinking significantly increases the risk of stomach cancers, a weakening of the heart muscle, atrophy of a number of nerve cells in several areas of the brain—particularly those dealing with memory and coordination. The earlier one starts heavy drinking the more significant are the effects on the body.

In drinking to the point of drunkenness, one will incur a substantial number of small brain hemorrhages and an even larger number of plugged brain capillaries. Around each of these points some brain cells will die for lack of oxygen. Research on brain cells indicates that apparently our bodies cannot rebuild new brain cells as we can other types of body cells. (But it should be noted here that recent research at U.C.L.A. suggests that perhaps some brain cell regeneration may be possible.)

The average adult brain contains about 17 billion cells, so the destruction of even a few thousand cells in a single drinking bout leaves the drinker with thinking abilities apparently in tact. However, years of drinking show an accumulation of scars caused by the hemorrhages. Autopsies of heavy drinkers show many areas of brain atrophy where the brain cells have been destroyed. Entire convolutions (large folds) of the cerebral cortex have been shown to be shrunken.

In a study of adolescent monkeys, done at the Scripps Research Institute in California, monkeys were given citrus flavored alcohol drinks an hour a day for 11 months. This would be equivalent to an hour a day of binge drinking. Two months later they were killed and their brains analyzed. It was found that their brains had 50 to 90% fewer stem cells in hippocampus compared to the control group. The hippocampus is involved in both short and long-term memory and spatial navigation. (5)

Absorption of alcohol occurs in the body through the tongue, stomach and small intestine. It can be slowed if the drinker has consumed a full dinner. High protein foods stay in the stomach longer and slow down the absorption of the alcohol into the bloodstream by as much as 50%. The Alcohol Safety Action Project of Phoenix, Arizona recommends that hosts and hostesses planning to serve alcoholic drinks at parties serve a combination of high protein foods during the party, such as: meats, cheeses, chicken livers, sea foods, hard boiled eggs, or sour cream dips.

The absorption of alcohol can also be speeded up. Carbonation, which increases the speed with which the alcohol enters the small intestine, is a factor in increasing the speed of intoxication. Therefore, champagnes, carbonated wines or liquors mixed with soda, tonic, or carbonated soft drinks speed up absorption and intoxication. Another factor which can speed alcohol absorption is the emotional set of the drinker. A person who is nervous may secrete more stomach acid. This acid can increase one's ability to absorb the alcohol quickly.

Once absorbed into the blood, the liver begins to convert the alcohol into water and carbon dioxide. However, it is not done quite that simply. One of the products in the breakdown of the alcohol in the liver is acetaldehyde -- which is more toxic than alcohol. The acetaldehyde is then attacked by the enzyme, acetaldehyde dehydrogenase, and another substance called glutathione, which contains high quantities of cysteine (a substance that is attracted to acetaldehyde). The acetaldehyde dehydrogenase and the glutathione form the nontoxic acetate (similar to vinegar) which deactivates the acetaldehyde and stops its damaging action.

However, the liver's stores of glutathione are quickly exhausted so if several drinks are ingested in a few hours, the acetaldehyde will not be deactivated and will do its damage for a relatively long time. The hangover is one of the more obvious manifestations of this damage. The damage of the acetaldehyde in heavy drinkers may be one of the factors in the development of the disease cirrhosis of the liver which is the bane of heavy drinkers. There is definitely a heavy toll on the liver when it is forced to oxidize large amounts of alcohol over long periods of time.

The "Hangover" effect, which often results from drinking, may be caused by several factors. The alcohol and other ingredients in the drinks may contribute to the unpleasant feelings called "hangovers." Alcohol distends (widens) the blood vessels of the brain. Distended blood vessels are a cause of many types of headaches. Another factor, as mentioned above, is that as the alcohol breaks down into acetaldehyde. The toxicity of the accumulating acetaldehyde causes general body disturbances such as headaches and nausea. Since the liver oxidizes alcohol at the rate of 1/4 to 3/4 of an ounce per hour the headache will eventually pass away. The metabolism of alcohol can be speeded up somewhat by ingesting fruit sugars (fructose) which is found in honey and fresh fruit and juices. This can be done before or after imbibing.

The headache may be eased by drinking coffee. The caffeine constricts the blood vessels. One might also sit up in a dark room for a few hours. Lying down, however, would increase the flow of blood to the head. A cold compress applied to the head might also decrease blood flow.

The analgesic characteristics of aspirin may also help to relieve the headache. However, since alcohol and aspirin combined cause a chemical reaction which disintegrates the stomach lining it is not wise to take aspirin until the alcohol has left the stomach and has entered the small intestine. This might occur within twenty minutes if the stomach was empty before drinking, but might be a few hours if the stomach was full of food while the drinks were being ingested.

The dry mouth that often occurs after drinking is a result of the dehydration of the body which occurs as the alcohol is being metabolized. One might drink lots of water, but juices and salt would be better. Salt and other minerals lost through the increase in urination also need to be replaced. Chicken soup or beef broth are very good sources of these minerals.

The congeners (flavoring and coloring agents added to alcohol) are also thought to be responsible for the effects of hangover. Light colored liquors, such as white wine, vodka and gin are low in congeners, so should reduce the severity of a hangover. Dark liquors such as red wine, brandy, rum and whiskies are high in congeners and would, therefore, increase the effects of hangover.

Alcohol as a preventer of heart disease has been suggested by a number of studies recently. Red wine has been touted as being particularly beneficial in increasing the good cholesterol (HDL). The major factor seems to be resveratrol, a powerful anti-oxidant. (Resveratrol can be purchased as a dietary supplement. Normally there is as much of the antioxidants in one pill as in a whole bottle of red wine.) So while it is true that red wine, in particular, and alcohol generally may have a positive effect on preventing some heart attacks, it is not the whole story. The studies that prompted the findings compared Italy, France, and the United States, as well as some other European countries. It is true that the French and the Italians drink far more red wine than do Americans and have fewer heart attacks. However they also die from alcohol caused diseases far more than Americans. Cirrhosis of the liver and esophageal cancer are three times higher among the French than the Americans.

The southern Europeans have some other dietary differences than the Americans. They eat much less red meat. They eat more fruits and vegetables. And they consume more fiber in their diets.

Some of the negative factors of increased alcohol consumption include: more calories added to the diet--which may increase one's weight-- and higher blood pressure due to the alcohol. Both of these are risk factors for heart problems. A greater chance for depression to occur, and an increased rate of accidents on the job and on the highway are also considerations. These are in addition to the increased risk for cancers such as mouth, esophagus, stomach, liver, intestinal, pancreatic, breast, and prostate. However for some reasons moderate drinkers live longer than non-drinkers.

The effects of alcohol on behavior are determined, to a large degree, by what the person expects to happen or wants to happen. While alcohol depresses the ability of the brain to function normally the behaviors which the individuals exhibit may be quite varied. One person may fight, another may sleep, one may become very outgoing, another over-amorous. So we find that inhibitions are usually relaxed.

Alcohol probably affects people by decreasing the amount of oxygen that the brain can utilize. A lack of oxygen in pilots has the same effect. At 9,000 feet (without supplemental oxygen) one can become "high" or drunk.

WHY PEOPLE DRINK

"I enjoy the taste, " is a reason often given for one's taste for alcoholic beverages. It seems that connoisseurs are usually certain that their favorite beverages are preferred because of the taste. This premise may be open to some question. Studies at California Polytechnic University, however, found that beer drinkers were unable to identify "their favorite beer" when they could not see it in the bottle. Scotch and bourbon drinkers were unable to tell the difference between the expensive and the inexpensive brands. And wine drinkers could tell red from white wines but could not differentiate between the cheap and the expensive varieties. The real reasons for preferring alcoholic beverages is more likely to be related to unconscious adjustments that we make to problems and unconscious needs which have not been fulfilled.

In a study funded by the National Institute of Mental Health (5) it was determined that the primary motivation for abusing alcohol is the unfulfilled power needs of people. The typical reasons for drinking usually given, such as: "to reduce anxiety, " "I like the taste," or "If I drink I can put things off" were not nearly as important as the inferiority complex brought about by unfulfilled power needs.

The study found that strong, but unfulfilled, power drives often turn people to alcohol, yet the alcoholic consumption reduces one's power drive and makes it less likely that such drives will be fulfilled. It was found that heavy drinkers could usually be predicted by their need for dominance. Among the factors that may be responsible for a greater need for power are: a weak physical body build, aging, an insufficient masculine self image (machismo), an insufficient feminine self image, insecurity with the opposite sex, and poor childhood experiences.

Psychologist Sharon Wilsnack of the Harvard Medical School has found that women tend to drink to feel more womanly. The alcoholic woman finds that drinking makes her feel more warm, loving, sexy, pretty, and considerate. However, the descent into alcoholism makes her neglect her appearance, decreases her ability to cope with life, and increases the disapproval of society that she feels. All of these make her feel less womanly. It was also found that women alcoholics gave more masculine answers to tests on sex role styles than did nonalcoholic women.

Another reason for drinking was theorized as a result of the studies done at Silver Hill Foundation in New Canaan, New Jersey. Their findings indicated that perhaps the alcoholic is "over-civilized. " That is, alcoholics tend to be overly conscientious, guilt ridden, hard workers and loaded with feelings that they cannot express--such as anger, sadness or love. The alcoholics who were studied drank to escape from the pressures of their lives, not because they wanted to derive pleasure from their drinking.

The Silver Hill study found that alcoholic housewives tended to be perfectionists. They were compulsive about being orderly. They couldn't tolerate dirty dishes in the sink or dirty clothes in the hamper. And outside of the house they were hard workers in organizations.

DRINKING AND DRUNKENNESS

The amount of alcohol a person can drink is determined, to a large degree, by one's body weight. The greater the volume of blood in the person, the greater the amount of alcohol that can be dissolved in it. Also, larger people generally have larger livers with which to oxidize the alcohol. So it is the alcoholic content of the blood, not the total number of drinks, that determines one's degree of drunkenness.

100% alcohol is considered 200 proof. So a 90 proof whiskey is 45% alcohol. And a 12% wine is 24 proof. The chart gives an idea of the amount of alcohol one might expect in blood if a given number of drinks were consumed in one hour. The amount of blood alcohol decreases as the weight of the drinker is increased. Note that not all drinks contain the same amount of alcohol. A 12 ounce bottle of malt liquor has twice the alcohol of an average bottle of beer. A martini has twice the alcohol of a highball. Even in beers there is a considerable difference in alcoholic content. Michelob contains the most alcohol by volume (5. 71%) compared to Lite's low of 4.34%. And, of course, a 100 proof liquor contains 10% more alcohol than an 80 proof liquor.

The blood-alcohol level is expressed in milligrams of alcohol per deciliter (mg/dL) of water or blood. Using this measure, 100 mg/dL is equal to one tenth of one percent alcohol in the blood. Consequently, 100 mg/dL would be equal to a 0.1% concentration. This level is above the allowable level in nearly every country in the world. In all states, 80 mg/dL (0.08) represents the threshold concentration above which a person is legally drunk when operating a motor vehicle.

Blood Alcohol Level Effect On Body

0.02 Slight mood changes

0.06 Lowered inhibition, impaired judgment, decreased rational decision-making abilities.

0.08 Legally drunk. Deterioration of reaction time and control.

0.15 Impaired balance, movement, and coordination. Difficulty standing, walking, talking.

0.20 Decreased pain and sensation. Erratic emotions.

0.30 Diminished reflexes. Semi-consciousness.

0.40 Loss of consciousness. Very limited reflexes. Anesthetic effects.

0.50 Death. Death has occurred at 0.35.

While the simplest guideline to remember if you are driving in the U.S. is that for each drink consumed, wait at least one hour before driving--and proportionately a longer time for smaller people.

If a person has been drinking for several hours, just divide the number of hours into the number of drinks plus one, to find the blood alcohol content. For example, if a 120 pound (55 kg) person has had 11 drinks in a four hour period, add one to the number of drinks (to allow for slow absorption of the first drink). We now have 12 drinks, divided by 4 hours. This is equal to 3 drinks per hour. The 120 pound person would have a blood alcohol level of approximately 0.094 and would be legally drunk everywhere in the world.

The US has one of the most lenient levels for determining whether one is legally drunk (0.8). Levels at 0.0 such as in Hungary or 0.02 in Norway indicate that America is not in the mainstream relative to drinking and driving.

A recent study done at the University of California, San Diego, found that having a blood level of alcohol of just 0.01 increases the chances of a serious traffic accident. Analyzing the data from 1994 to 2008 from fatal car accidents were 36% more severe when even a barely detectable amount of alcohol (0.01) was in a driver's blood. The researchers also found that the more alcohol the person had, the more likely they were to drive fast.(7)

HOW MUCH IS TOO MUCH?

Various groups have set different criteria for determining what is moderate, heavy, and alcoholic drinking. The most lenient proposal today is one drink a day for women and two drinks for men. However some advocate not drinking daily and others place the maximum at one drink a day. There is always a trade-off when drinking, even moderately. For example, while the chance of a stroke caused by thrombus may be reduced by moderate drinking, the chance of a stroke due to the bleeding caused by a ruptured aneurysm is increased. There is also the question of genetics. Some people have the genetic tendency toward a number of diseases with even small amounts of alcohol. Yet others have genetic strengths against the damage alcohol. It is wise to look at those in your extended family to see if drinking may have caused problems, including alcoholism.

ADDICTION TO ALCOHOL

The late Father Joseph Martin, perhaps the country's most respected speaker on alcoholism, himself an alcoholic, said that "If alcohol causes problems--it is one." This may be the simplest yet most complete definition of alcoholism. Whether or not there is a physical addiction, we might well define drinking as a problem when it affects one's job, one's relationships or negatively affects any area of one's life.

What we would call the abuse of alcohol occurs when someone continues drinking after there have been problems caused by alcohol such as driving drunk, missing work or relational problems.

The Diagnostic and Statistical Manual of Mental Disorders, 4th edition, defines alcohol abuse as drinking despite alcohol-related physical, social, psychological, or occupational problems, or drinking in dangerous situations, such as while driving. The World Health Organization's International Classification of Diseases refers to "harmful use" of alcohol, or drinking that causes either physical or mental damage in the absence of alcohol dependence.

SIGNS OF ALCOHOLISM

Drinking in secret, to keep others from knowing how much is being drunk.
Overriding concern with drinking. Drinking becomes more important than people.
Drinking the first few drinks fast to "get high" quickly.
Development of guilt feelings because of the drinking:
Avoids talking about alcohol, usually for fear that the excess drinking will be criticized.
Rationalizes drinking behavior; one can always give a reason for drinking (to celebrate, to drown his sorrows, because it is Friday).
Often tries to protect one's ego by being important, leaving large tips, buying drinks for strangers, etc.
Often feels remorse from the guilt about drinking.
May observe periods of total abstinence to prove that one really doesn't need alcohol. The alcoholic wants to leave the impression that it is possible to "take it or leave it. "
May change drinking patterns. Changing the types of drinks or the times or places which had been usual occasions for drinking.
In extreme cases the alcoholic may neglect everything except drinking and may become very introverted.

Financial problems or shame may affect the family of the alcoholic making them withdraw from normal social situations.
Hiding bottles of liquor so that the supply will not run out.
Alcoholics may feel a great deal of self pity or resentment because of imaginary injustices they have suffered.
Nutrition is often neglected in favor of drinking.
Sex drive decreases. This sometimes makes alcoholics accuse their spouse of infidelity.
Morning drinking.
Drinking to avoid the withdrawal symptoms. Since alcohol can be an addicting "downer" the absence of alcohol can develop such symptoms as shaking and hallucinations in the alcoholic.
Drinking during working hours and missing work because of alcohol.

Lessening of tolerance for alcohol. Since the liver loses its ability to oxidize alcohol as liver tissue is destroyed by the alcohol, the alcohol stays in the body longer. It, therefore, takes less alcohol to get drunk and the effects of the alcohol are increased and prolonged.

Brain damage, loss of memory and personality changes.

Last night at twelve I felt immense,
But now I feel like thirty cents. . . .

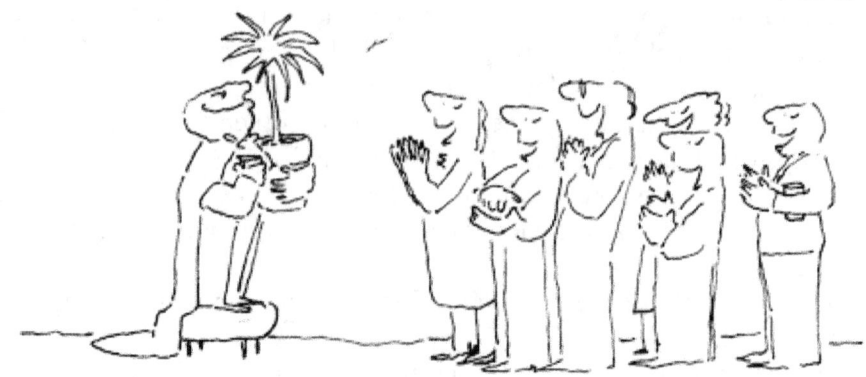

There is some evidence to suggest that some alcohol addiction and opium addiction are caused by the same chemical, tetrahydropapaveroline (THP). THP is the chemical in the opium poppies from which morphine is made. It is formed in the brain when acetaldehyde (a breakdown product of alcohol) combines with the byproducts of certain body enzymes and dopamine.

Genetics may play another part in addictions. Some combinations of genes may increase the amount of pleasure from a drug or make withdrawal from a drug more painful. Another combination of genes may give one person a painful experience while another gets pleasure from the same drug. For example, an element of a dopamine receptor gene (DRD2) is more common with people addicted to alcohol or cocaine.

Studies with mice give us some interesting insights—and question! One study pinpointed a gene that makes withdrawal from depressants less severe. Another found a gene that reduced the mouse's response to morphine. Another showed that those with a lack of a serotonin receptor were more attracted to alcohol and cocaine. There are a number of such studies showing that certain genes increase or decrease one's rewards from various drugs.(8)

Not all alcoholics are physically dependent on alcohol. Such dependence is diagnosed when the body craves alcohol and when increased amounts of the drug are required in order to achieve the desired euphoria. If a person can stop drinking for a week without having convulsions, tremors or hallucinations it is a sign that the person was not physically addicted to the drug. But all alcoholics are mentally "habituated" to the drug. That is, their minds need alcohol in order to adjust to the problems that surround them.

If a person is physically addicted to alcohol the safest procedure is to hospitalize the patient. A doctor can then administer either alcohol or preferably a short acting barbiturate that has depressant properties similar to alcohol. By decreasing the dosages gradually it is often possible to gradually detoxify the alcoholic while keeping the withdrawal symptoms to a minimum.

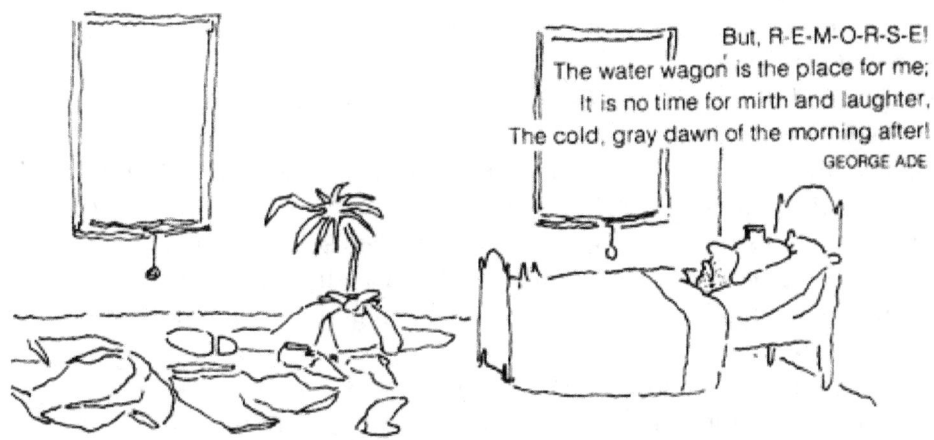

But, R-E-M-O-R-S-E!
The water wagon is the place for me;
It is no time for mirth and laughter,
The cold, gray dawn of the morning after!

GEORGE ADE

Alcoholics Anonymous uses the following questions to determine whether or not a serious problem exists. If you answer yes to four or more of the questions you either have a serious drinking problem or you may have one in the future:

1. Have you ever tried to stop drinking for a week or longer only to fall short of your goal?

2. Do you resent the advice of others who try to get you to stop drinking?

3. Have you ever tried to control your drinking by switching from one alcoholic beverage to another?

4. Have you ever taken a morning drink during the past year?

5. Do you envy people who drink without getting into trouble?

6. Has your drinking problem become progressively more serious during the past year?

7. Has your drinking created problems at home?

8. At social affairs where drinking is limited, do you try to obtain extra drinks?

9. Despite evidence to the contrary, have you continued to assert that you can stop drinking on your own whenever you wish?

10. During the past year, have you missed time from work as a result of drinking?

11. Have you ever blacked out during your drinking?

12. Have you ever felt you could do more with your life if you did not drink?

TREATMENT FOR ALCOHOLISM

Alcoholism usually ends in one of several ways. The brain functions may completely disintegrate so that the alcoholic must be institutionalized for life. The alcoholic may die. Or the alcoholic finds that the rationalization system which has been used to justify the excessive drinking finally breaks down. The alcoholic may then seek help.

Quite often it is a traumatic event, such as a divorce, loss of job, or jail that makes the person realize the degree to which alcohol has influenced one's behavior and one's life. Commonly people who are deeply interested in the recovery of the alcoholic, or another drug dependent person, will set up a "confrontation." The confrontation is designed to break down the rationalization system of the drug dependent person. In a one to one conversation the drug dependent person will deny and rationalize his or her behavior. In the confrontation, which is done with professional help, a number of the family, friends and coworkers are assembled. When the drug dependent person attempts to deny or rationalize previous behavior, there is always someone who can confront the denier with the truth. Very often an effective confrontation will stimulate the person to honestly seek treatment.

Once this happens and the alcoholic admits to the seriousness of the problem it is possible to treat the disease. While there is some conflict relative to whether or not an alcoholic can take another drink, most evidence suggests that a recovering alcoholic cannot take another drink.

In the last half century there has been a move to recognize alcoholism as a disease or an abnormal adjustment pattern rather than a moral flaw or a criminal activity. Yet quite often when people under treatment for alcoholism relapse by taking a drink, the treating institution throws them out and refuses further treatment. But refusing to treat someone because that person exhibits a symptom of illness seems unique to the problem of alcoholism. When a depressed psychotic is sad, when an ulcer patient exhibits intestinal pain, or when an asthmatic child has difficulty in breathing, they are treated rather than rebuked.

The major types of therapy available to alcoholics are: avoidance therapy, professional psychotherapy, and the voluntary "self help" groups.

A common type of avoidance therapy uses the drug Antabuse (disulfiram) which blocks the effects of alcohol by interfering with the breakdown of acetaldehyde by blocking the effect of acetaldehyde dehydrogenase--which was mentioned earlier in the discussion of hangovers. As long as the alcoholic takes the Antabuse pills there should be no desire to drink because the negative affects far outweigh any positive effects. And since the drug remains in the blood for several days, an alcoholic cannot suddenly stop the pill and immediately indulge in a sudden impulse to drink.

The problem with this technique is that while it may take away the undesirable adjustment pattern, the alcoholic still has problems and a need to adjust to them. Some type of psychotherapy is therefore often needed to help the alcoholic to find new methods of problem solving and adjustment.

Sometimes psychotherapy, either group or individual therapy, can be used to assist the alcoholic to find a way out of the disease. Hypnosis is sometimes used along with other therapeutic methods to aid in modifying the unhealthy behavior.

The therapy that has helped the most alcoholics is the Alcoholics Anonymous approach. If the individual recognizes that it is a problem and can accept the assumptions of the group it can be highly successful. The major assumption of the organization is that one must place one's faith in a higher power to overcome the problem. Another important part of the therapy is that a member can always call on another member for support if a problem develops and the urge to take a drink becomes too great. This and other related behaviors can help to satisfy one's need to love and be loved.

THINGS TO THINKS ABOUT!

--We learn to tolerate nearly everything if given or taken in excess -- abuse, cruelty, war, poverty.

--We crave excitement and fulfillment. Is it in the real world of living, thinking and feeling--or is it contained inside a gelatin capsule or the smoke of a weed ?

--The greater our unhappiness, the greater our need to escape.

--We substitute one thing for another: sex for love; alcohol for success; and methadone for heroin--how often do we delude ourselves.

--You pay for cocaine the same way you take it--through the nose.

--"Cocaine amplifies your personality. But what if you're an ass?" Bill Cosby

WHERE TO GO FOR HELP

Addicts Anonymous, http://www.alladdictsanonymous.org/

Alcoholism and Drug Addiction Treatment Center 800-477-3447 (Information and referrals)

American Council for Drug Education 301-294-0600 (Representatives will discuss drug issues and find help for callers): http://www.acde.org/

Cocaine Anonymous. (213) 839-1141 http://www.ca.org/

National Clearinghouse for Alcohol and Drug Information. (800) 729-6687,(301) 468-2600. http://www.higheredcenter.org/resources/national-clearinghouse-alcohol-and-drug-information-ncadi Box 2345, Rockville, Md. 20852. (Free printed material and audio-visual material)

National Cocaine Hotline (800) COCAINE

National Council on Alcoholism and Drug Dependence Hotline 800-475- HOPE http://www.ncadd.org/

National Drug Information Center of Families in Action. (404) 934-6364, (Coordinates parents groups and matches callers with local services)

http://www.nationalfamilies.org/

National Institute for Drug Abuse 800-662-HELP, Spanish 800-66-AYUDA

http://www.nida.nih.gov/nidahome.html

Mothers Against Drunk Driving http://www.madd.org/

Alcoholics Anonymous

475 Riverside Dr

New York, NY 10115

(212) 870-3400

Local offices will be listed in your phone book

Al-Anon Family Group Headquarters

Box 862 Midtown Station

New York, NY 10018

(800) 356-9996

Local offices will be listed in your phone book

The BACCHUS and GAMMA Peer Education Network

Box 100430

Denver, CO 80250-0430

(303) 871-3068

Materials and programs geared toward college students

National Clearinghouse for Alcohol and Drug Information

Box 2345

Rockville, MD 20847-2345

(800) 729-6686

National Institute on Alcohol Abuse and Alcoholism

National Institutes of Health

US Department of Health and Human Services

6000 Executive Blvd

Bethesda, MD 20892-7003

(301) 443-3860

END NOTES

Volker A. Coenen, Thomas E. Schlaepfer, Burkhard Maedler, Jaak Panksepp. Cross-species affective functions of the medial forebrain bundle—Implications for the treatment of affective pain and depression in humans☆. Neuroscience & Biobehavioral Reviews, 2010.

Gingras, J.L. (1990). Maternal cocaine addiction. Medical Hypotheses, 33(4), 231-234.

3. Fusar-Poli P, Crippa JA, Bhattacharyya S, et al. (January 2009). "Distinct effects of {delta}9-tetrahydrocannabinol and cannabidiol on neural activation during emotional processing". Archives of General Psychiatry 66 (1): 95–105.

4. Science Daily, February 3, 2009: Manzar Ashtari, Kelly Cervellione, John Cottone, Babak A. Ardekani, Sanjiv Kumra. Diffusion abnormalities in adolescents and young adults with a history of heavy cannabis use. Journal of Psychiatric Research, 2009; 43 (3): 189-204.

5. Taffe, MA. Long-lasting reduction in hippocampal neurogenesis by alcohol consumption in adolescent nonhuman primates. Proceedings of the National Academy of Sciences. June 1, 2010.

6. Reported in the book The Drinking Man, by McClelland, et al.

7. Phillips DP and Brewer KM. The relationship between serious injury and blood-alcohol concentration (BAC) in fatal motor vehicle accidents. Addiction, 106: 2011

8.. http://learn.genetics.utah.edu/content/addiction accessed October 24, 2011

CHAPTER 12
PHYSICAL FITNESS

Why should I exercise when I am older?
Is stretching daily enough exercise?
What is the best exercise for me to do?
How much walking is enough exercise?
Here are some answers—

Fitness means that the individual is able to perform the normal daily activities with adequate energy and still have the vigor to perform additional activities. If a person can finish the daily chores of work, housekeeping, or weeding, and return home with the energy necessary to play tennis, jog, or work on a hobby, a minimal level of fitness has been achieved. The higher one's level of fitness, the greater will be the reserve of energy throughout the day. As we age our physical fitness often suffers because we don't keep working at it.

The physical effects of exercising for endurance (aerobic fitness) are many. It benefits every body organ. The major emphases of exercise have correctly been focused on the benefits to the heart and circulatory system. But it should be noted that the bones and ligaments, digestive and excretory systems, the lymphatic and respiratory systems all benefit.

The well-conditioned person not only is able to ward off infectious diseases and cancers better than the poorly conditioned person (because of a more effective immune system), but the chances of developing heart disease, strokes, diabetes, and other types of degenerative and chronic diseases are also lessened.

The mental effects of exercise have long been observed by athletes and physiologists of exercise. People exercising regularly generally have shown higher than average levels of social maturity, self-confidence, and intellectual efficiency. The question is--did the athletic activity actually develop these qualities or were they already present in the person and perhaps were instrumental in the decision to become an athlete?

A study at Purdue University showed that untrained middle-aged university employees significantly improved their mental outlooks during the duration of a specially-designed fitness program of calisthenics and jogging. Results of the study showed that statistically-significant positive changes had occurred. The areas of self-assurance, stability, and imagination were all greatly improved in the test subjects. A number of studies have shown reductions in depression even in neurotic patients. If the exercise is sufficiently long and intensive a "high" from the flood of endorphins (natural brain opioids) can happen. Lesser amounts of exercise can reduce some negative effects of stresses. And of course if the exercise is also "fun" it is natural that depression will be reduced or eliminated. Enjoyable forms of exercise might be golf, tennis, skiing or jogging through the woods, or whatever you find enjoyable. There are, of course, many recreational activities that are enjoyable but are not really effective exercise, such as: bowling, chess, shuffleboard, croquet and yoga. They too may be valuable in reducing stress, which might also reduce one's blood pressure.

The circulation of blood to the brain during exercise aids in making one more alert. The physical activity during an exercise can also allow one to take out aggressions on inanimate objects, becoming more relaxed in the process. When people hit a tennis ball or pound the pavement while jogging, they may be unconsciously taking out frustrations that otherwise be directed at a boss, a spouse or a neighbor.

There is a substance called catecholamine that is essential in several brain chemicals which help to transmit messages in the brain. One of the essential precursors for this brain chemical is called tyrosine hydroxylase (TH). TH decreases with age and may be a factor in mental changes and problems that can occur with age. The Geriatric Research, Education and Clinical Center of the Department of Veterans Affairs Medical Center in

Gainesville, Florida has done a study with rats which showed that exercise reduced the loss of TH. If this checks out with humans we may have yet another reason for mental benefits of endurance exercise. (1)

Another reason for exercising aerobically is that we look better when we exercise effectively. And when we look good, we feel good. This aesthetic value of exercise, usually combined with some diet changes, is a reason that we see so many people of all ages exercising before the summer beach season.

The benefits of exercise to a society and its economy have been recognized by the governments of China, Japan, and Russia. In those countries "exercise breaks" often take the place of coffee or tea breaks. Many U. S. companies are developing exercise programs to increase the physical and mental health of their employees and to increase their longevity. Such programs have been shown to increase job performance by making the people less prone to make errors, more able to produce, and less likely to miss work.

A number of people participate in Masters competition. This competition usually begins in the 30 to 40 year age range and can go to 100. There are competitions in running, swimming, orienteering, rowing, cycling, volleyball and nearly every other sport one can imagine. In a Canadian study on masters' participants during the seven year follow up of the 750 respondents (aged 40 to 81 with an average of 58), far fewer than expected had developed a serious illness over the 7 year study. Most had given up smoking before or during their training period. Only 2.9% still smoked while 32.8% were former smokers. The participants were shown to have been more interested in their health than the general population, as shown by their increased use of seat belts when driving and a greater propensity to see a doctor if something seemed wrong. And more important, their outlooks are happier and their lives seem more fulfilling.

The advantages of exercise apply equally to women and men. The old notions that exercise was un-feminine have long been dispelled. The fascinatingly feminine Olga Korbut of the Russian gymnastic team captured the hearts of the world in the 1972 Olympics. Then Nadia Comaneci of Romania did it again in 1976. Then Florence Griffith-Joyner of the U.S.A., the Olympic sprint champion in 1988, did it. Caroline Wozniaki the number one ranked Danish tennis player or T'erea Brown the American sprinter in the 2012 Olympics are among the huge list of world class athletes..

In fact women champions in every field have shown the advantages of physical fitness. It has finally been recognized by the medical profession and the Olympic Committee that women can do anything that men can do. This idea has filtered to the general population where we now see women running, lifting weights, playing soccer, and water polo and boxing in addition to the sports they have traditionally done--swimming, tennis, gymnastics, and riding.

The fears of some, that women who exercise would become too muscular, have proven unfounded. The fact is that exercise aids in slimming the figure to conform to the bone structure of the natural female anatomy. Exercise can flatten the abdomen, remove excess fat, firm the muscles, and assist in the development of a more attractive posture. Proper exercise can also aid in shaping the body to more desirable dimensions.

It is now recognized that women, because of their larger fat stores, can have greater endurance than can men. The marathon is a 26 mile 385 yard (42.2km) race. Women continue to reduce the time margin between them and the faster men. However in the super-marathon events women's times generally equal men's times by the time they have run 35 to 43 miles (56 to 70 km). They then generally become faster than the men. This is probably due to lighter body weight, more fat stores, and a better ability to convert fat into sugars for energy according to studies at the University of Cape Town. (2)

A study in Minnesota of 40,000 women, aged 55 to 69, showed that as little as one day a week of exercise significantly reduced their death rates. But the more physical activity they got, and the more vigorous it was, the lower their death rates. (3) Good physical condition can aid women in reducing most of the diseases of aging.

Exercise also aids in relieving the menstrual discomforts which are often experienced. The high body heat and the increased circulation, which occurs during exercise, aid in relieving the congestion of blood in the uterus, a major cause of discomfort.

A Harvard University study found that female runners produced a less potent form of estrogen than did their non-exercising counterparts. This was held to be a factor in the 50% reduction of expected cases of breast and cervical cancers and a 65% reduction in a type of diabetes that is more common among women than men.

Age is a factor in choosing the types and amounts of exercise which one should do. A person who has been exercising regularly will be "younger" than a person who has not been exercising. That is, the condition of the person's body, its biological age, will be less than that expected for that person's chronological age. So while for the average person their conditioning level (scientifically called the VO_2 max) reduces about 1% per year after age 25, a well conditioned person can slow or even reverse that normal condition of aging. Staying fit can cut that figure in half or even reverse it. (4)

If someone has not done much exercise, the body may appear older than it is. The bones can be softer, the blood pressure higher, the amount of artery hardening greater, the blood supply less, the digestive processes slower, the muscle cells reduced through degeneration, and many other such factors which we associate with age can be present. But if that same person were to begin an effective exercise program, those results of aging can be slowed, stopped, or even reversed.

Osteoporosis (porous bones) an affliction of many older women and some thin men, can be prevented or reversed by weight bearing exercise. Walking or running, weight lifting, or calisthenics can all prevent its development. Swimming, while an effective endurance exercise, does not prevent the disease because the water, not the person's body, supports the body's weight.

People can continue to exercise throughout their lives. Evidence indicates that such exercise should help to prolong life because it keeps the body younger. A few years ago, a San Francisco man made headlines. He was over 100-years-old but he ran seven miles each day--on his way to work as a waiter. When he finally retired from that job, at 103, he took a job working in a gym.

You may have heard of the Abkasian peasants in the U. S. S. R. who live to be very old. Their longevity is attributed to their exercise. Not long ago, one of the boys from this area was accepted into medical school. After his graduation, he took his mother to live with him in the city, thinking that she deserved a rest in her old age. Although she had been healthy when she arrived, her health failed rapidly in the city. When she returned to the farm and working in the fields, her health returned to normal.

Exercise can make you feel better and live longer, no matter when you begin your program. If you begin when you are young and continue the program, you may add years to your life--and life to your years. But you are never too old to begin. After all, exercise may be the next best thing to the fountain of youth.

The elements of physical fitness should be understood by anyone considering pursuing an effective path toward fitness. These elements are:

. Flexibility - the ability to move the joints of the body through a wide range of motion.

· Strength - the ability to lift a weight one time.

· Endurance or stamina - the ability to perform a certain task for a long period of time.

· Agility - the ability of the body to exhibit coordinated muscular movements.

Everyone should possess a minimum acceptable level of endurance, adequate strength to live their chosen lifestyle, and sufficient flexibility to be able to move freely and to have an acceptably good posture.

CARDIO-VASCULAR ENDURANCE

Endurance (stamina) is the ability of the body to continue work or exercise over a long period of time. Stamina is developed by exercises which make the heart beat fast—particularly when it is at least 30 minutes. This is the most important aspect of physical fitness.

Most of us have the minimum level of flexibility and strength to live our lives effectively. We generally have enough sugar in our blood or fat on our bodies to give us fuel for energy. However, we often lack the ability to exercise at a level beyond that which is our norm.

Those who have developed cardio-vascular (heart-blood) or cardio-pulminary (heart-lung) endurance have trained their bodies to use oxygen efficiently. Since oxygen is just as important in developing energy as is blood sugar but cannot be stored like sugar, the ability to use oxygen effectively must be developed.

Very few people function at even the most minimal fitness levels. Yet proper exercise, for as little as 30 minutes each day, can make one's body function better, control obesity, reduce mental tensions, and reduce one's chances of heart and blood circulation problems. For one's physical and mental health, for a better chance at a longer and happier life, there is probably no better investment of one's time than in a daily dose of proper endurance exercise.

Most national medical associations have now taken the position that, "Exercise is the most significant factor contributing to the health of the individual." Study after study indicates that proper endurance exercise is a major factor in increasing one's chances of living a longer life. A study of over 17, 000 British executives showed that those who exercised vigorously had only one-third the risk of developing a fatal disease during middle age than light exercisers or non-exercisers.

The effects of endurance exercise on the circulatory system are:

--The heart enlarges, enabling it to pump more blood in less time to the muscles and tissues that need it. The enlarged heart beats slower than a normal heart when resting; it has a longer rest period between each beat.

--The red blood cells become more numerous. These are the cells which carry oxygen from the lungs to the muscles and other tissues of the body. The increase in these blood cells enables each beat of the heart to carry more oxygen to the tissues.

--The number of blood vessels being used in the muscles is increased. This gives the muscles more capacity for using the oxygen which is brought to them in the blood.

The heart is really a double pump. One pump (the right heart) receives "used" blood which has just come from the body after delivering nutrients and oxygen to the body tissues. The blood is received into the right atrium (Latin for room). It is then pumped into the right ventricle where the next heart beat pumps this dark, bluish red blood to the lungs where the blood gets rid of a waste gas (carbon dioxide) and picks up a fresh supply of oxygen which turns it a bright red again. The second pump (the left heart) receives this "reconditioned" blood from the lungs in the left atrium. The next beat pushes the newly oxygenated blood into the heavily muscled left ventricle. The next beat pumps the blood out through the great trunk-artery (aorta) to be distributed by smaller arteries to all parts of the body.

The heart can enlarge normally, because it has been forced to work hard to pump the blood of a person who exercises for long periods of time. Swimmers, basketball players, and long distance runners usually have such enlarged hearts. This "normal" enlargement is generally considered to be good.

Abnormal heart enlargement is found in many people for various reasons. These people's hearts have been forced to beat rapidly for reasons other than exercise. The heart of an obese person will have to beat many more times each day just to pump blood through the excess fat of that person. Some people have abnormally enlarged hearts because their heart valves do not function efficiently. Many have abnormally enlarged hearts because their arteries are clogged and narrowed so the heart must push the blood at a much higher pressure to get the blood to the organs and muscles. The previously mentioned heart valve damage can also cause the heart to enlarge due to the extra work that it is forced to do.

A normally enlarged heart will beat slower than normal as it enlarges. An abnormally enlarged heart will generally continue to beat relatively fast since it has enlarged because of extreme stresses. Its enlargement would allow more blood to be pumped with each beat. But because of the great demands of the body (such as in obesity) or in the heart's inefficiency (such as in damaged valves), enlargement is not enough. The heart must therefore continue to beat at a relatively fast rate.

The pulse rate is the number of heart beats per minute. The average heart beats 70 to 80 times per minute when the person is at rest. But the lower the pulse rate, the better conditioned the person is. Some athletes have pulse rates in the 30's. A pulse rate of 50 would be very good for the average person. A former Swedish tennis great had a pulse rate of 28. This was achieved because of the way he practiced, continually running while hitting for several hours every day.

There are several methods of finding your pulse rate. First you must find an artery which is near to the skin. The most common places are: just inside the muscle on the left side of the neck ; at the base of the neck just inside the collar bone, on the inside of the wrist about two inches below the base of the thumb, or directly over the heart. Place the fingers, not the thumb, of one hand on one of these spots. If your fingers are at the correct place, you will feel a throbbing. Each throb is a pulsation of blood from the heart. Count the number of beats for one minute. Or, count the number of beats for 15 seconds and multiply by four. This will give you your resting pulse rate in beats per minute. If you are exercising you might count for six seconds then multiply by 10 to get your pulse rate.

A heart which beats 70 beats per minute has one-half second to fill with blood. This resting phase is called the diastolic period. If the pulse rate is increased to 120 beats per minute the resting phase is reduced to one-fourth of a second. In spite of the shorter resting phase, the heart still remains functional to about 160 beats per minute. At that point the resting phase may be so short that the right atrium of the heart cannot fill completely with blood, and each beat may pump less blood.

jEven though the resting phase of the heart is diminished, there are other things which happen to keep the heart efficient. The blood pressure increases, which pushes more blood into the heart. The veins may be being massaged by the muscles as the muscles contract, which aids in the more rapid return of blood to the heart. The blood becomes more acidic due to the lactic acid formed in the muscles as a result of the use of sugars for energy. This acidic quality makes the hemoglobin in the red blood cells more able to pick up the oxygen in the lungs. These factors enable the heart to pump four to ten times as much blood during heavy exercise as during rest.

The well-conditioned person's heart gets more resting periods than does the heart of the person in average condition. If a person's heart were to beat 20 times less per minute (i. e., 60 rather than 80 beats per minute), it would save nearly 10, 000 beats during a night's sleep and nearly 30, 000 beats in a 24-hour day. It would get 18 days per year more rest than the heart with the higher pulse rate.

The heart is a very strong pump. Each day it pumps about 13 tons of blood. Each minute it pumps the total volume of the body's blood through the circulatory system. During heavy exercise, it may pump the entire volume of the blood of the body nine times each minute. That's a lot of work for a 12-ounce organ.

Red blood cells carry the oxygen from the lungs to the body tissues, by means of an iron compound called hemoglobin. These red blood cells are 1/3500 of an inch in diameter. They are formed in the bone marrow and live about three months. When red cells are destroyed, the body reclaims most of the iron and uses it to form new red cells. If one's diet is deficient in iron, it will probably result in anemia. (a lack of red cells.)

The more blood and red cells present in each unit of blood, the greater the oxygen-carrying capacity of the blood. If a person lives high above sea level, the body's need for oxygen increases. This is because the air at high altitudes is less dense, so there is less oxygen per cubic foot of air. The body then manufactures more red blood cells so that a greater proportion of the oxygen in the air is absorbed. The Aymara Indians of the Andes Mountains have an average red cell blood count of 8 million per cubic centimeter of blood. The average person at sea level has a red cell count of about 4. 5 million. Strenuous exercise and high altitude living both have the same effect on the red cell count. As the body's need for oxygen increases, the red blood cells increase to accommodate that need--if the diet contains sufficient iron..

Exercise also increases the total amount of blood in the body. The average person can increase the total amount of blood by 10 to 20 per cent during ten weeks of effective endurance training. This can increase the blood volume by up to two quarts. Well-trained athletes may have over 40 per cent more blood circulating in their bodies than do average people. This means that the heart doesn't have to pump as often to get the needed oxygen to the muscles and other tissues because each spoonful of blood carries more red cells and consequently more oxygen.

The condition of the muscles is another factor in one's endurance. Only the muscles which are specifically involved in the activity gain endurance. The legs of a long distance runner or cyclist, and the chest and upper back muscles of a swimmer will have developed changes when they become well-conditioned. The number of small blood vessels (capillaries) being used by the muscle will increase so that more blood will be able to circulate through the muscle. This allows more oxygen and blood sugars to be available for energy.

HOW MUCH EXERCISE DO I NEED?

The original work of Dr. Ken Cooper in his book titled "Aerobics" required several exercise sessions each week at a fairly high level of intensity. Later the American College of Sports Medicine adopted and refined a more stringent program. However the work of Dr. Steven Blair, of Dr. Cooper's Institute for Aerobic Research in Texas, indicates that if your objective for exercising is merely living longer, you can exercise at a lower level of intensity. Dr. Blair has used research based on 25,000 people followed for many years to develop his theory.

The "minimal exercise requirement" allows a person to build up his or her exercise during a day. The ''maximum fitness exercise program'' requires a person to do 20 to 30 minutes work at one session to achieve maximum results. Dr. Blair's minimum requirement would allow a person to add the exercise done in a day to achieve the minimum 30 minutes. So, if you walk 10 minutes in the morning, climb stairs for a total of 1 minute during the day, garden for 20 minutes, then ride a bicycle for ten minutes in the evening you would have totaled at least 41 minutes of exercise during the day. Just 30 minutes is enough to increase your chances of living longer. (5)

Dr. Blair's analyses of his 25,000 subjects over the years has led to a large number of scientific articles and has changed our thinking relative to what is a minimal work out for extending our life spans.

On the other side of the exercise spectrum, work at Dr. Cooper's Center indicates that if you exercise with some intensity, which is the message of this book, you need not exercise more than a half hour in order to get many of the benefits necessary for maximum heart disease protection. Exercising up to 60 minutes per day gives additional benefits. More than 60 minutes a day at a high pulse rate does not seem to reduce the risk of heart disease. More than 60 minutes would burn more calories and contribute to weight loss. It would also reduce the risk of some types of diabetes. However the wear and tear on the joints from running might be a negative risk factor for too much jogging. So more than an hour a day of exercise should only be done if it is enjoyable and does not cause any physical pain. (6)

A British study indicates that you need to burn 7.5 calories per hour in order to gain improved health. (7) suggests a weekly output of 2,000 calories in exercise in order to achieve a minimal level of fitness. This would require five hours of exercise per week with an expenditure of 8 calories per minute.

So to determine how much you should exercise depends on what do you want.

--If you want to extend your life some and feel better, do 30 minutes of increased exercise each day—not necessarily continuously;

--If you want a higher level of fitness with a greatly lessened heart attack risk do 30 minutes of continuous exercise at 65 to 90% of your maximal heart rate. (220 minus your age).

--If you want still more benefits exercise up to an hour at the higher heart rate.

--If you want to lose fat exercise longer but at a much lower pulse rate.

EXERCISING FOR BETTER AEROBIC FITNESS

Effective aerobic exercise, according to The American College of Sports Medicine (ACSM) report of 1990, requires that aerobic exercise be done 3-5 times per week for 20-60 minutes each session at an intensity of 60-90% of maximum heart rate or 50-85% of maximal oxygen consumption. (In addition, ACSM recommends the inclusion of a strength training program 2 or 3 days a week, flexibility exercise and coordination activities for overall health benefits.) (8)

To determine your target heart rate zone (where your heart rate should be while exercising to increase cardiorespiratory fitness), you must first determine your maximal heart rate. This is done by subtracting your age from 220. Then, you can determine the limits of your intensity by multiplying your maximal heart rate by between .6 and .9. (The higher number is for better conditioned people.) For instance, if you are 50 years old, then your maximal heart rate is 220 - 50 = 170. To determine your minimal target heart rate, multiply 170 x .6 = 102 beats per minute. For the top of your target heart rate zone, multiply 170 x .9 = 153 beats per minute. Beginners should begin at the low end of the target heart rate range, and slowly increase their exercising heart rate as their body adapts to the increased physical demands of exercise.

Physiologists use another measure to determine cardiorespiratory fitness

The VO_2 max is the major physiological measurement used by exercise physiologists. It determines the amount of oxygen that a body can use to develop energy while exercising. (The maximum amount of oxygen used (VO_2 max) is the number of milliliters (ml) of oxygen (O_2) per kilogram of body weight per minute.)

Males generally have about a 20% higher average VO_2 max than females. Age also influences it. A 20 year old male will probably average 50, a 40 year old will probably drop to 40, and a 70 year old to 30. The highest numbers recorded are 96 for a man—the Norwegian cross-country skier, Bjørn Dæhlie—world and Olympic champion and 78 for Joan Benoit, Olympic marathon gold medal winner.

While you will never get to that 96 level of conditioning you can certainly improve your own level through exercise.

How about you?

To determine your maximal oxygen consumption rate (VO_2 max), you can do the Rockport Fitness Walking Test (9) This has been validated by ACSM as an appropriate fitness test.

The Rockport Walking Test

In the test you will walk a mile then immediately count your heart rate (pulse rate). You will then check the accompanying charts to find your fitness.

To take the test--

Find a flat measured quarter mile track. Or measure a course. (You might drive your car a mile on a road then mark the one mile distance.

Warm up by walking a few hundred yards at a leisurely pace.

With a stop watch, or a watch with a second hand, note the time you started.

Walk briskly for an exact mile. Walk as fast as possible for the mile.

Note the time you took in minutes and seconds. __:____

Immediately count your pulse rate for 15 seconds then multiply it by 4 to get your pulse per minute. You can put your finger on the opposite wrist, just above the thumb or feel the pulse in the side of your neck under the muscle about two inches below your ear, or just put your hand over your heart.

(Number of heart beats for 15 seconds)_____ x 4 =_____ Pulse rate per minute)

Measuring your VO_2 max through the Rockport Fitness Walking Test

1. Your time for the mile walk (from number 5 above).___(minutes):____(seconds)

2. Convert the seconds to hundredths of a minute. ____

(For instance, if your walk time was 10 minutes, 15 seconds = 10.25. This is the number you will plug into the following formulas.(ie. Divide the number of seconds by 60.)

3. Use the following gender-specific formulas to determine maximal oxygen consumption rates (VO_2 max).

Male

_____ = 0.0947 x ____ (your body weight)

_____ = 0.3709 x ____ (your age)

_____ = 3.9744 x ____ (your mile time)

_____ = 0.1847 x____ pulse rate after the mile (from number 6 in previous list.)

_____ Total points

Take 154.899 and subtract the above total to determine your VO_2 max.

154.899 - _____ (total points)= _____ Your VO_2 max

MEN--HOW DO YOU RATE?

Rating /Age	30-39	40-49	50-59	60+
Superior	>49.4	>48	>45.3	>44.2
Excellent	45-49.4	43.8-48	41-45.3	36.5-44.2
Good	41-44.9	39-43.7	35.8-40.9	32.3-36.4
Fair	35.5-40.9	33.6-38.9	31-35.7	26.1-32.2
Poor	31.5-35.4	30.2-33.5	26.1-30.9	20.5-26
Very Poor	<31.5	<30.2	<26.1	<20.5

Men's 1 mile walk fitness score

Men rated in the highest 1/3 of fitness have a 39% lower risk of heart disease and stroke than those in the lowest 1/3. Additionally, premature deaths can be reduced by almost half if one just gets out of the "poor" category.

Female

_____ = 0.0585 x ____ (your body weight)

_____ = 0.3885 x ____ (your age)

_____ = 2.7961 x ____ your mile time (in minutes and hundredths of a minute) From number 2 above.

_____ = 0.1109 x ____ (mile heart rate pulse rate after the mile--from number 6 in previous list.)

_____ Total points

Take 116.579 and subtract the above total to determine your VO2 max.

116.579 - _____ (total points) = _____ Your VO_2 max

WOMEN--HOW DO YOU RATE?

Rating /Age	30-39	40-49	50-59	60+
Superior	>40	>36.9	>35.7	>31.4
Excellent	35.7-40	32.9-36.9	31.5-35.7	30.3-31.4
Good	31.5-35.6	29-32.8	27-31.4	24.5-30.2
Fair	27-31.4	24.5-28.9	22.8-26.9	20.2-24.4
Poor	22.8-26-9	21-24.4	20.2-22.7	17.5-20.1
Very Poor	<22.8	<21	<20.2	<17.5

Ladies 1 mile walk fitness score

Ladies in their 40s with a VO_2 Max lower than 24.5 (Poor) have nearly a 40% greater chance of developing diabetes.

Now that you know your maximal oxygen consumption, you can test to see if your cardiorespiratory fitness program is working by occasionally repeating the above test. As your fitness level increases, your VO2 max will increase because cardiorespiratory fitness relies on the effective delivery and use of oxygen to make energy.

TO BEGIN A CARDIOVASCULAR FITNESS PROGRAM

If you are in poor or average condition and desire to increase your fitness level, be sure that you begin with a low intensity activity such as walking or use a low intensity level on a stationary bike or a stair climber. Whichever approach you take, start slowly. If you begin any exercise program too quickly, you will probably have some muscle soreness for the first few days. This soreness discourages some people, but it will disappear and will probably never return as you get into condition and keep fit. Any exercise caused muscle soreness will peak in two days and be completely gone in 5 to 7 days.

Keep improving by increasing the amount of time spent exercising and/or the intensity at which you exercise. Eventually you will reach your fitness objectives. When you reach these objectives, you can continue to work at that level for maintenance.

Just about any time is a good time to exercise. However, if you exercise just before you go to bed, you will increase your metabolism, which may make it more difficult to sleep. If you exercise just after eating, you will force your body to divide the available blood between the stomach, which needs it for digestion, and the skeletal muscles, which need it for exercise. But if you exercise just before a meal time you may find that you don't desire as much food. If you use your exercise sessions to give you energy, you may choose to exercise in the morning. If you use your exercise sessions to relieve the stress and tension of your day, the evening would be a more appropriate time.

Endurance exercise requires a proper warm up, a vigorous activity period, and a cool down session. Even well-conditioned people often show abnormal electrocardiograms when they exercise without a proper warm up. However they will show normal electrocardiograms when they are "warmed up" prior to exercising. A warm up is designed to increase blood flow to the muscles you are going to work. So, a brisk walk would be an appropriate warm up to a jog, and a few minutes on a rowing machine or a slow swim would get the blood flowing to your upper body before a swimming workout. You can also perform the activity you plan to engage in for your workout at a very light intensity for a proper warm up. A good indication that you are properly warmed up is when you begin to sweat. Five minutes is usually sufficient to get your body ready for your workout.

There are different reasons to stretch before or after a workout. If you want to increase your flexibility you would definitely want to stretch after your workout. However stretching before a workout may set you up for injuries.. Research is finding that runners tend to have more injuries if they stretch than if they don't. Swimmers don't swim as fast if they have stretched. Stretching cold muscles increases your chance of injury, so if you do want to stretch before you work out it is better to stretch after you are warmed up. If you are trying to increase your flexibility, you may choose to stretch after your cool down, as your muscles are guaranteed to be warmed up after your intensive workout. In fact, stretching after exercise is more important than stretching before in terms of increasing your flexibility.

Cooling down after an exercise period is important if the exercise has been vigorous. It is suggested that the activity be slowed until the heart rate has reached a rate of about 100 beats per minute. When a person stops immediately after exercising, a great deal of blood may pool in the veins which may decrease the amount of blood available to the brain. If a person does not cool down properly, dizziness or fainting is possible-- shock is a remote possibility, and even a heart attack is possible.

The best endurance exercises include: cross country skiing, running, swimming, aerobics, stair climbing, cycling, rowing as well as walking on a treadmill or exercising on a bicycle exerciser. The worst endurance exercises for cardiorespiratory fitness are weight lifting, calisthenics, archery, horseshoes, and bowling as these are of no use in developing endurance.

Sports can be a vehicle to becoming better fit. Handball, squash, soccer and basketball are vigorous enough to qualify as endurance exercise if played continuously for a long period of time.

Most sports require some amount of athletic ability and many assist one in developing some amount of strength, flexibility, and endurance. But the major benefit of most sports is that they allow us to relax while being active. Sports, especially the hitting sports, such as tennis and badminton, or the body contact sports, such as football or basketball, can be great stress relievers. Of course, some people get "up tight" about winning which may do more mental harm than good. If you like to compete, most countries now have ''master'' sports programs which encourage participation or competition in your favorite sport.

MAKE IT FUN

Effective exercise is going to make you feel better physically and mentally. This will happen whether you enjoy the exercise or not. But why not enjoy it? If you live in a cold part of the country you can cross country ski. If you enjoy swimming -- swim. If you like to run -- run. If you like to play basketball -- play. If you like to dance -- dance. It doesn't matter if it is ballet, country western, swing or jazz, as long as your heart rate is increased. Anything that you do physically will help a little. Walk up the stairs at work. Take a walk while you talk at lunch.

If you like outdoor activities run or walk your way to fitness. These are the most common approaches to exercise. Many people are now enjoying orienteering. If you join an orienteering club you will take your map and run from point to point as the map requires. So your brain must work along with your legs. Orienteering is becoming more and more popular. There are now national and international competitions.

Running, stair climbing, or cycling may be boring for you. If so, you might try to make it entertaining by playing music in your headset with you while you jog. Or you might watch television or read while you exercise indoors on some form of stationary aerobic equipment. Try to do something to make exercise enjoyable for you, because the benefits you receive from it are well worth the effort!

Working in a health studio environment is enjoyable for many people. You can lift weights with friends, ride the exercise bike in front of the TV or watch a movie, take an aerobics class, or take a ''spinning'' class. In ''spinning'' the class works with an instructor. All are on exercise bikes. With the music the instructors pedals forward or backward, fast or slow and the class mimics the instructor's movements.

Some of us like to work at home because it doesn't take any commuting time to go to the gym. You can jump rope, follow an aerobics program on TV, or ride the exercise bike while watching TV or reading. If you want to read you can buy a commercially made book holder which attaches to the bike's handlebars—or you can rummage around the local hardware store and make your own with plastic, clamps and tape.

If you are not already exercising effectively, are you motivated to look and feel better and to live longer? How strong is your motivation? You now have the knowledge necessary to begin an effective exercise program. Has it changed your attitude? Will it change your behavior?

When it comes to running for fun Sir Roger Bannister may have said it best.

"We run, not because we think it is doing us good, but because we enjoy it and cannot help ourselves. The more restricted our society and work become, the more necessary it will be to find some outlet for this craving for freedom. No one can say, 'You must not run faster than this, or jump higher than that.' The human spirit is indomitable."

SOME MORE STUFF
TYPES OF MASTERS' COMPETITION AT THE WORLD GAMES
Alpine skiing (slalom, giant slalom, Super G)
Badminton (singles, doubles, mixed doubles)
Basketball
Biathlon
Bowling (singles, doubles, team)
Broomball
Cross country skiing (30K men, 20K women, freestyle men 15, 50 K, women 10K and 30K
Curling
Mixed curling
Darts (singles, doubles, team)
Diving
Figure Skating (ice dancing, precision skating,
Handball (4 wall)
Ice hockey
Indoor archery
Indoor athletics (track and field) 50m. To 5000m, 10K, 50m hurdles, 1500 and 5000m walk, high jump, long jump, shot, triple jump, pentathlon
Indoor shooting (pistol and rifle)
Indoor soccer
Indoor tennis (singles, doubles, mixed doubles)
Judo
Racquetball
Ringette
Snooker/billiards
Speed skating (both short and long tracks)
Squash
Swimming
Synchronized swimming
Table tennis
Team handball
Triathlon
Volleyball
Water Polo (from men aged 30)
Weightlifting
Wheelchair basketball

Sledge hockey

General age group rule (some exceptions)
Men's groups (from 35) 35-39, 40-44, 45-49, 50-54, 55-59, etc.
 Women's groups (from 30) 30-34, 35-39, 40-44, etc
 Disabled 25 and up (one category).

Benefits of aerobic exercise
An increase in the number of blood vessels. When this occurs in the heart, it increases one's chances of avoiding or surviving a heart attack.
Control of body fat. One-half hour of proper exercise daily will keep off (or take off) 26 pounds per year.
An increase in the basal metabolism for several hours after exercising, which may take off additional pounds.
An increase in HDLs (the good blood cholesterols).
A strengthening of the diaphragm, the major muscle used in breathing.
An improved immunity system to fight off degenerative and infectious diseases.
Stronger bones and connective tissue.
A reduction in minor aches, pains, stiffness, and soreness.
Increase productivity.
A reduction in chronic fatigue.
An increased ability to relax and to sleep well.
An increase in endorphins in the brain (if the exercise is sufficiently long), making one feel exhilarated.
Improved digestion and bowel function.
Increased mental capabilities (i.e. increased alertness) due to an increase in oxygen to the brain.
Increased muscle tone.
Increased self-esteem.
Increased creativity and imagination.
Decreased muscle tension and stress.
Decreased PMS symptoms and menstrual cramps.
Decreased labor pain and faster recovery time from giving birth.
Lower resting heart rate from a larger stroke volume.
Lower resting blood pressure.
Increased life expectancy and better quality of life.
Wonder how many calories you're using?
 Calories x Weight x Number = Total calories
  per hour   in lbs   of hours   used

Sleeping or lying in bed. 0.12 x _____ x _____ = _____
Sitting (reading, computer
 bathing, eating, etc.) 0.17 x _____ x _____ = _____

Standing (washing, shaving,
cooking, etc.) 0.26 x _____ x _____ = _____

Light work (housework, driving,
 mechanic, slow walking) 0.38 x _____ x _____ = _____

Faster work (table tennis,
 volleyball, sailing or canoeing,
 golf) 0.55 x _____ x _____ = _____

Heavier manual labor (carpenter,
machine operation, plumbing,
shoveling snow) 0.64 x _____ x _____ = _____

Active sports (downhill skiing,
tennis, badminton, dancing,
fast walking, slow jogging) 0.77 x _____ x _____ = _____

Very heavy exercise (cross country
skiing, running fast, basketball,
football, digging, sawing with
hand saw) 0.90 x _____ x _____ = _____

Total calories used in a day _____

How many hours in the week did you use 480 calories (minimum for fitness)

_____

Minimal fitness level by walking. It need not be continuous, but is cumulative
throughout the day.
Women--Walk 2 miles in under 30 minutes at least three days a week.
OR, 2 miles in 30 to 40 minutes 6 or 7 days a week.
Men--Walk 2 miles in under 27 minutes at least 3 days a week,
OR, Walk 2 miles in between 30 and 40 minutes 6 to 7 days per week.

END NOTES

Tumer N, LaRochelle JS, Yurekli M ''Exercise training reverses the age-related
decline in tyrosine hydroxylase expression in rat hypothalamus,'' J Gerontol A Biol Sci
Med Sci 1997 Sep; 52(5): pp255-259.

Bam, J. Et al. ''Could women outrun men in ultramarathon races?'' Medical Science
in Sports and Exercise. Vol. 29 No. 2. 1997. Pp. 244-247

Kushi, L.H. Journal of American Medical Assn. 1997. Vol. 277. Pp. 1287-1292

Klissouras, V. "Aerobic Power in Old Humans: Genes and Environment." World
Congress of Sports Medicine, Orlando, FL. May 31, 1998.

Blair, S.N. et al. ''Influences of cardiorespiratory fitness and other precursors on
cardiovascular disease and all-cause mortality in men and women.'' Journal of the
American Medical Association 276:205-210, 1996

Blair, S. "Physical Activity, Fitness and Health: An Overview." Presentation at the
World Congress of Sports Medicine, Orlando, FL. June 2, 1998

Morris, J.N. et al. Exercise in leisure time. British Heart Journal. 1990. 63:pp 325-
334) An American study (Paffenbarger, R. S. Et al. ''Some interrelationships of physical
activity, physiological fitness, health and longevity.'' In Bouchard, C. Et all. Physical
Activity in Fitness and Health. Champaign, IL. Human Kinetics, 1993. Pp. 119-133

American College of Sport Medicine. New guidelines for quantity and quality of
exercise. Medicine & Science in Sports & Exercise, July 2011.

Kline, Porcari, Hintermeister, Freedson, Ward, McCarron, Ross, and Rippe, 1987

CHAPTER 13
GAINING STRENGTH

The American College of Sports Medicine, while primarily interested in aerobic activity as a producer of health, has added strength training, flexibility and coordination as ideal elements of physical fitness. Each adds an important factor in feeling better and living longer. Strength training not only strengthens the muscles and bones but it makes us better able to carry on our daily duties. Flexibility allows us to move the same ranges of motion that we did when we were younger. Aging tends to tighten our connective tissue, like our ligaments and tendons, so it is well to keep them stretched. Coordination tends to reduce as we age, especially as we get elderly. Often the cerebellum, an important part of the brain, loses some of its ability to aid us in balancing.

The National Institute on Aging, Gerontology Research Center has done a 25 year study on aging men and women and the loss of strength and power (power a combination of speed and strength). At about age 40 both strength and power declined in both sexes. However power declined faster than strength in men. (1) With the loss of muscle cells and the reduction of physical work we can expect that strength will decrease. But many of us want to keep that loss minimal by exercising for strength and power.

The amount of strength one needs depends on the type of occupation and recreational activities he or she performs. Both men and women need some strength. A female truck driver needs more strength in her job than does a male secretary. She can gain the necessary strength needed by doing the proper exercises. But everyone needs some strength activity to keep the bones and muscles from becoming weaker. Yes, the bones degenerate if they are not forced to support weight and porous bones (osteoporosis) can result.

There are four types of strength exercises:

-- Concentric (isotonic) or dynamic exercises in which the muscle moves a joint through a certain range of motion--pushing the body upward in a push up or jumping up would be examples of concentric exercises;

-- Isometric exercises in which the muscle contracts but does not move the joint-- examples would be holding an object without moving it or standing in a doorway and pushing out on the door jamb;

--Eccentric contractions are those in which the muscle is lengthening rather than shortening during the exercise-- an example would be lowering the body back to the floor during a push up or landing on the ground after jumping upward;

--Plyometric exercise is a combination of the eccentric then concentric contractions are rapidly performed--and example would be landing from a jump then rebounding into another jump.

Any one of these types of muscle contractions can aid you in gaining strength. However the most commonly used is the concentric exercise. If you were trying to gain strength in your wrist to be able to serve a tennis ball better you would do a concentric exercise moving your wrist through a full range of motion.

There are two major factors that affect one's strength-- the number of muscle fibers contracting at one time and the efficiency of the lever (joint and muscle attachments). A muscle is made up of thousands of small muscle fibers, each one about the size of a straight pin. Not all of the fibers in a muscle will contract at the same time, but every fiber contracting will do so in its maximum ability. This is known as the "all or none" principle. The greater percentage of fibers which a person can make contract at one time, the greater the force which can be exerted.

Every joint is a lever which varies in efficiency. The biceps muscle in the front of the upper arm works on a more efficient lever than does the calf muscle (gastrocnemius), which allows one to rise up on the toes. And levers also vary in efficiency from person to person. Those who have shorter bones generally have better lever actions than those with longer bones. Heavily-muscled people generally have more efficient levers, as well as more muscle fibers, than do the tall thin people. This why you don't see tall thin competitors in Olympic weight lifting events.

The American College of Sports Medicine lists use recommendations for resistance exercise:

Adults should train each major muscle group two or three days each week using a variety of exercises and equipment.

Very light or light intensity is best for older persons or previously sedentary adults starting exercise.

Two to four sets of each exercise will help adults improve strength and power.

For each exercise, 8-12 repetitions improve strength and power, 10-15 repetitions improve strength in middle-age and older persons starting exercise, and 15-20 repetitions improve muscular endurance.

Adults should wait at least 48 hours between resistance training sessions.

It might be noted that one set of repetitions can give 90% of the strength gain that three sets can give. So if you short of time one set of each exercise will suffice. The key is that you exhaust your muscle on each exercise. Your muscles will not adjust much in gaining strength unless they are forced to their maximum.

While the ideal method of gaining strength is by the use of heavy resistance apparatus, such as is provided by barbells and dumbbells, it is possible to gain strength by using one's body as the resistance for the muscles. The following exercises do not require apparatus:

1. For the front of the chest (upper pectorals) and the back of the upper arms (triceps), do push ups. If you cannot do a regular push up, the resistance can be reduced by keeping your knees on the floor or by pushing away from a wall.

2. For the front of the upper arms (biceps), lie on the floor. Bend your legs while keeping your feet flat on the floor, lock your hands behind your thigh, and pull your head

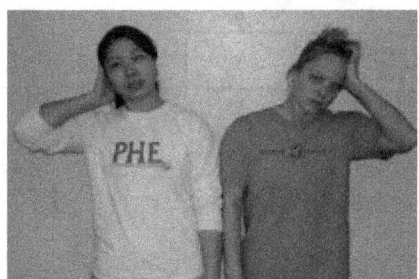

and shoulders up to the knees. This exercise will also stretch the back muscles. Another exercise for the biceps is to use your other hand to give you resistance while you bend your arm.

3. For the forearms, squeeze a tennis ball or push one hard against the other. You can also lift a broom with your wrist. As you become stronger, move your grip farther from the bristles of the broom--or get a heavier broom. Who knows, you might even work up to lifting a shovel. This broom exercise is particularly good for strengthening the wrist for a tennis serve if you hold the broom palm up and for the golf swing if it is held palm down..

4. For the neck, put your hand on your head (the front, back or side, depending on which muscles you wish to strengthen). Push the head against the hand. With pressure on the back of the head it will help to correct the postural defect of a "forward head."

5. For the upper leg, steady yourself by holding on to a table. Do a one-legged half knee bend. Do not let the upper leg go past the position at which it is parallel to the floor. Connective tissue in the knee may be damaged if you do a full knee bend. If you are not strong enough to do a one-legged knee bend, do the exercise with both legs. By doing the exercise with one leg rather than two, you double the amount of weight which the leg muscles are forced to lift. This is good for skiing and running.

6. For lower leg, steady yourself by holding on to a table, then rise up on your toes. Do this one leg at a time. This is good for running.

7. Lifting any weight over your head will also put some stress on the vertebrae of your spine and help to prevent osteoporosis.

If you can do the exercises more than 12 times, you need more resistance if they are to be the most effective strength exercises.

RESISTANCE TRAINING FOR STRENGTH

The most common exercises done in gyms generally involve at least two muscle groups acting at the same time. For example, the bench press and the pushup both use the upper chest muscles and the back of the upper arms. It is impossible to determine just how much each muscle group is working when these exercises are done.

For example, if two people do push-ups, one may be doing fifty-five per cent of the work with the chest muscles and forty-five per cent with the triceps (the muscles in the back of the upper arm) Another person may be doing far more of the pushing with the triceps than the chest muscles.

For general strength conditioning, the exercises which use two muscle groups are fine. However if you are a person who wants to develop each muscle to its greatest strength, it would be best to isolate the muscles you desire to develop. Competitive athletes are the people most likely to desire such optimum strength development. However, if you were a skier you might well concentrate on the muscles in the front of your thighs because they often tire first. A golfer might want to concentrate on wrist or rotary abdominal strength.

There are two criteria for finding the best exercise for any muscle. First, the muscle group for which strength is to be developed should be isolated from other muscle groups so that only that muscle is involved in the exercise. Second, the joint involved in the exercise should be exercised through the greatest range of motion possible. By doing this, the muscle and the connective tissue associated with that muscle will be stretched to the maximum. This gives the person maximum flexibility for that joint while still achieving maximum strength.

Another factor important in determining the greatest development of strength is that the muscle should be exercised until it is exhausted. This exhaustion should occur at about eight to twelve repetitions of the exercise. If you can do ten repetitions, the weight is probably too light for maximum strength development. However if you don't need maximum strength just do 12 to 15 repetitions. Anything helps.

DO SAFE EXERCISES

Since there are some exercises which may damage tissue, they should be avoided. The previously-mentioned deep knee bend or "squat" is one. If a person does a full deep knee bend, the ligaments in the front of the knee begin to be stretched after the leg has been bent more than 90 degrees. If a person continues the knee bend to the point where the calf muscles and the muscles at the back of the thigh touch, the stretching of the knee ligaments is greatly increased. So while a deep knee bend would strengthen the muscles that work the knee, it would weaken the internal structure of the knee joint. For most people this may not be a great problem, but for those who play golf, tennis or who ski, it can make the knee more susceptible to being sprained.

Any potentially-harmful exercise that stretches the connective tissue in the abdominal area by bending too far back, should be avoided. It is desirable to have tight connective tissue in the abdominal area to assist the muscles in supporting the visceral organs in the abdomen.

Another dangerous exercise is one that puts great pressure on the discs of the lower spine. The "dead lift," in which one bends at the waist and lifts a heavy weight with the lower back muscles, is such an exercise. This exercise can put as much as 3,000 to 5,000 pounds of pressure per square inch on the lower spinal discs. Such pressure has ruptured the discs of some weight lifters. It can also weaken the discs and make them more susceptible to injury later in life.

Pulling forward on the neck, which was common in the older style of sit ups is also contraindicated because it may stretch the connective tissues in the back of the cervical vertebrae.

The exercises that adhere to the above criteria--isolation of the muscle, maximum flexibility of the joint, and little chance of damage to the body--are illustrated in the weight-lifting photos. Remember that as soon as you can do 10 to 12 repetitions, you can add more weight for your next workout. Remember too that as you ago you have lost some muscle fiber so that you will not have the same potential for strength at 50 as you had at 20.

DESIGNING YOUR WEIGHT TRAINING PROGRAM

You must first decide what it is that you want. Do you want to lose weight, to increase your muscle size, to get stronger, to become more aerobically fit, to rehabilitate a muscle after an accident or surgery, or to become better at a particular sport. If you want more strength, power, or larger muscles you would want to train with weights or other types of resistance.

The number of repetitionsis important.

--For strength use a heavy weight that you can do for only 1 to 3 repetitions before your muscles are exhausted. Repeat this several times during your workout. This type of workout may work more on the brain than on the muscles--teaching the brain to be able to contract a greater percentage of muscle fibers, thereby increasing one's strength. Most of us at our age don't need maximum strength, but for those competing in master's level competition it may still be desirable.

--For hypertrophy (bigger muscles) exhaust your muscles in sets of 10 to 25 repetitions doing a total of 150 to 250 repetitions of the exercise during the workout. The continued repetitions increases the blood flow, increases the size of the connective tissue (tendons and tissues which hold the fibers together), as well as increasing the cross sectional size of the individual muscle fibers. Recent research also indicates that more muscle fibers may be developed. It was once thought that a person could not increase the number of fibers in a muscle. Hypertrophy seems to be better gained under eccentric work so lifting for one or two seconds then lowering for two to 4 seconds seems to work better.

--For muscle endurance use a very light weight and do the exercise 100 or more times. This brings more blood flow to the muscles and increases the number of slow twitch muscle fibers that can be utilized. Generally it is better to perform the activity for which you want the endurance, such as swimming, cycling, or running.

Breathing effectively while exercising is important to minimize the chance of hernia or of rupturing blood vessels while lifting heavy weights. The best method of breathing is to exhale while lifting the weight. The second best method is to inhale while lifting. Holding the breath is the most dangerous because the air pressure inside the chest cavity is increased when the muscles around the ribs and shoulders are contracting. This is called the Valsalva maneuver or Valsalva effect. The strain of the increased internal air pressure can push part of the intestine through the inguinal rings (holes) of the lower hip bone, causing an inguinal hernia.

DEVELOPING MUSCULAR ENDURANCE

It's not enough to have your heart healthy and more red blood cells. Your individual muscles also have to have specific endurance. The muscles you use in an endurance activity will develop a better capacity to use the oxygen and sugars which the blood brings to them. There will be more hemoglobin in the muscles, more readily available fuel, and there may even be a different type of muscle tissue developed.

There are three different types of muscle fibers, the slow twitch (red or type I), the intermediate (type IIa), and the fast twitch (white or type IIb). The fast twitch fibers are the strongest contract quickly but cannot do it for many repetitions. Olympic weight lifters have a high percentage of these because they need only one powerful contraction, then they rest for many minutes. Endurance athletes, such as cross country skiers, swimmers, and distance runners have a large percentage of the slow twitch fibers. These fibers contain more fuel and can contract many times. Alpine skiers are somewhere in between.

Research indicates that the type of training a person does can change the type of fibers present. It may be that it is the intermediate fibers that change more toward the fast or the slow twitch type of fiber.

INCREASING YOUR STRENGTH

Muscular endurance and muscular strength are at opposite ends of the spectrum. Strength is how much force can you generate in one muscular contraction while endurance is how long can you continue muscular contractions with relatively little resistance against them.

If you are a skier you never need the absolute maximum force that an Olympic weight lifter would need. But there are times when you need more than the normal amount of power. Your extra strength will even help you to get up after a fall. So there is a need for more strength at times. And when running or walking up a hill there is a need for more than the average amount of strength for a number of muscular contractions.

Your strength is determined primarily by the number of individual muscle fibers you can have contracting in one contraction. No one can contract all of the muscle fibers in a muscle at the same time. Few people can even contract 50% of their muscle fibers at one time. So your strength training program is designed to teach your brain to be able to contract more muscle fibers at one time.

The following exercises will help you to condition your muscles. If you are trying to get stronger exhaust your muscles in under 12 repetitions. Exhaustion in one to three repetitions is best. But if you are working on developing muscular endurance, such as you will use in making a long run, do a number of repetitions. You will be able to tell whether your are developing your muscular endurance by how your "quads" feel at the end of the day.

25 to 100 repetitions would be a good range for most people. But remember that your muscles should be exhausted when you finish. It is only by getting your muscles very tired that you will get the best results. However, remember that anything is better than nothing.

STRENGTH EXERCISES

1. THE ABDOMINAL CURL UP. The abdominals are important for posture, for running and any running sport, walking and skiing. Everyone knows this exercise but some have not kept up with the latest techniques to make it more effective. Lie on the floor, or on your bed:

--Put your hands on your chest (to avoid pulling in on the neck muscles),

--Bring your feet up as close to your hips as possible (so that you don't use the small hip flexing muscles which attach to the lower back--especially important for women),

--Look at the ceiling and continue looking at the same spot during the exercise (so that you don't stretch the muscles in the back of your neck), then

--Raise your shoulders and concentrate on bringing the lower part of your ribs closer to the top of your hips.

--Do as many repetitions as you can because you want muscular endurance from these muscles.

There are actually four sets of muscles in the abdominal wall. One, the *rectus abdominis*, does most of the work in the sit up. There are two sets of angled muscles called the "*obliques*." These also assist in the sit up but also work in twisting and sideward bending actions. The following exercises work on the "*obliques*."

146

2. THE TWISTING ABDOMINAL CURL UP is done the same as the above exercise but as you raise your shoulders you bring your right shoulder toward your left knee on one repetition, then your left shoulder to your right knee on the next one.

If you belong to a gym there may be a rotary abdominal machine, if so it is more effective than the twisting sit up.

Another exercise that can develop the abdominal obliques is the side sit up. Put your feet under a sofa or have someone hold them down, then, while on your side bring your shoulders and torso upward.

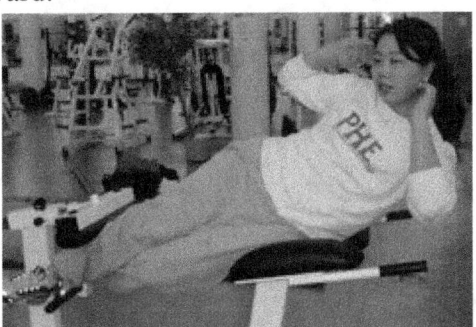

Another particularly good exercise is done lying on the floor on your back. Extend your legs straight over your hips. With your arms out to your side to keep your torso flat, allow your legs to come down to the right side, then bring them back up, then down to the left side.

SHOULDER EXTENSION is another important exercise for most people to do unless they have been swimmers or gymnasts—who use these muscles continually.. The upper back and back of the arm muscles are not used often but it is an important area to exercise when concerned with osteoporosis in the upper back.

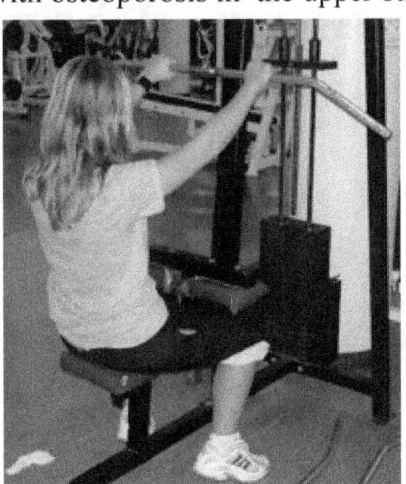

If you belong to a gym use a pull down pulley and pull it down with your arms straight. If you don't belong to a gym you can buy stretching bands at a sporting goods store or surgical tubing (about 8 to 10 feet) from a pharmacy. Screw an eye bolt into a door jamb or into a wall in the garage, anchor the middle of the band to the bolt. Tie knots in the end of the tubes, or make a handle, then pull--alternating arms or using both arms together.

THE TRICEPS (three heads) straighten (extend) the elbow. One of the three heads crosses the shoulder joint so it works with the "lats" in pulling the upper arm backwards. All three heads work to straighten the arm at the elbow joint.

If you belong to a gym use the triceps extension machine or do triceps extensions on the "lat" pull down machine. You can also raise a dumbbell over your head. If you don't belong to a gym you can do push ups with either your feet or your knees on the floor.

THE FRONT OF THE THIGH (quadriceps) helps you to run, walk, ski or cycle. It holds your leg in that bent leg position which is critical to downhill skiing. There is no question that these are the most important muscles for the alpine skier. You will want both muscular strength and muscular endurance in this group.

If you are in a gym use the quadriceps machine. If not, get a partner. Sit on a table. Have your partner place both hands on your ankle and give resistance. You straighten your leg. If you don't have a partner you can use that same rubber band which was recommended for the upper back.

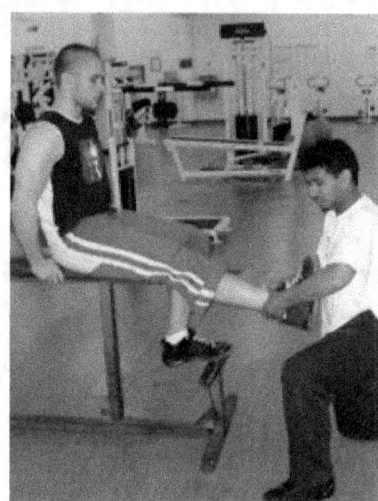

THE BACK OF THE THIGH (hamstrings) must be strong to counterbalance the quadriceps. Gyms have special machines for the hamstrings. If no machine, get your trusty old partner, lie face down on the floor or a table, and have your partner push against your ankle as you lift your lower leg from the floor. Keep the other knee on the floor.

THE BACK OF THE HIPS (gluteals) work in any walking, running, cycling or skiing action. They are also critical for posture. To get the upper part of the rear of the hips, the muscles that do a lot of your power work, with your quads, lie on a table face down with your hips on the table but your thighs past the table and your toes touching the floor. You can use a partner, if you want more strength, or do it alone, if you want more endurance by doing many repetitions. Start with one toe touching the floor while the other leg is brought as high as possible then alternate legs. This will look like an exaggerated kicking action for a person swimming the crawl stroke.

HIP AND KNEE EXTENSION gives you greater force potential from your hips and knees. Gyms all have either squat racks, sleds, or other machines which allow you to extend your legs. But it can be done easily at home. You can just do a 3/4 knee bend (don't bend your knees over 90 degrees) or you can do half knee bends. If you want twice the amount of resistance do your knee bends with only one leg. To do a half knee bend, hold a table top to steady yourself. Using only one leg bend down 45 to 90 degrees then return to a standing position. by doing it on only one leg you get the same effect as doing it with two legs while holding a barbell equal to your own weight.

CALF MUSCLES (*gastrocnemius*) are done by simply rising up on your toes then bringing your heels back to the ground. Repeat many times for endurance. If you want more strength, such as for hill climbing, balance yourself by holding a table or chair then do the exercise using only one leg at a time--the right leg until it is exhausted, then the left leg until it is exhausted.

HIP ABDUCTORS are those which move your legs sideways away from the mid-line of your body. They are very important in helping you to maintain your balance..

Some gyms have special machines for the abductors. If there is a "multi-hip" machine, use it. Most gyms have low pulley weights with ankle straps. Stand with one side of your body next to the machine and put the ankle strap on the leg farthest from the machine. Lift the leg sideways keeping it straight.

With a partner, lie on your side. Let your partner put pressure on your knee or ankle, then lift your leg as high as you can. If you have no partner you can do the same exercise alone--you just won't get as strong, but you can get just as much endurance.

You can also use the rubber bands. Attach one to a low part of a wall, hook your foot into a loop on the end of the band, and lift your leg outward.

HIP ADDUCTORS are those muscles high on the inside of your thighs. They also help in balancing. They also bring your legs back together if they have been moved outward by the abductors. The exercises are just the reverse of those for the abductors.

If your gym has a machine, use it. If there is a low pulley station stand sideways to the pulley but a yard away from the machine. Put the ankle strap on the ankle nearest the machine. Let your leg move outward (toward the machine) with the weight, then bring it back to the other leg.

With a partner lie on your back. Spread your legs. Let your partner give pressure inside you ankles. Bring your legs back together. If you wish, you can combine the adductor and abductor muscles in this exercise. While lying on your back your partner will give you hand pressure on the outside of both ankles. You will spread your legs against the pressure (abductors). Then your partner will give you pressure on the inside of your ankles and you will bring your legs back together (adductors).

Without a partner just sit on the floor with your feet about 12 inches from your hips and the heels together. Spread your knees outward, then grasp the inside of your knees with your hands. Bring your knees together as you resist the movement with your hands. You will feel the tension inside your upper thighs.

THE MUSCLES INSIDE AND OUTSIDE OF YOUR CALF also aid in balance. They should be strong enough to easily bring you back to a balanced position. The best way to work these muscles is to sit down, cross one leg over the other with your raised foot just past your other knee. Place one hand on the outside of the foot and move your foot outward as you resist with your hand. (The scientific name for this movement is "eversion.") Then put the other hand on the inside of the foot, near the ball of your foot, and resist as you bring your foot inwards (inversion).

LOWER BACK exercises should be more geared to muscular endurance than strength so you will want many repetitions. For most people it is the most important exercise which can be done because there are so many lower back problems related to muscular weakness. You can lie on the floor face down and lift your shoulders about 6 inches from the floor then return to the floor. (You don't want to go too high with your shoulders because you don't want to create a "sway back" in your exercise.

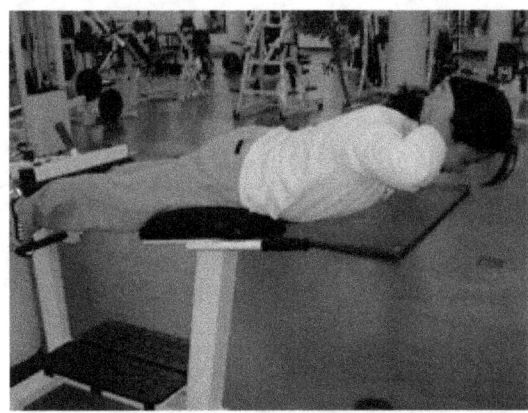

You can also do this with a partner. With the partner holding your legs, and your hips and legs on a table, bend forward at the waist to 60 or 90 degrees then lift your torso back up so that it is in line with your legs and hips. Again, you don't want to arch your back during the exercise.

HOW MANY REPETITIONS AND HOW MUCH WEIGHT you use depends on your goals. For pure strength you should be exhausted in 1 to 3 repetitions. But pure strength is not what you want for most activities. You want a certain amount of strength and you want muscular endurance. So you will want from 20 to over 100 repetitions. But anything you do will help.

Using a partner, using your own "manual resistance" can actually be better than using weights. Your partner can adjust the pressure to make you work to a maximum level on each repetition. Weights can't do this. Only partners and "isokinetic" machines have this capability. So if you are using a partner don't figure you are not getting the best strength work out. In fact that partner is probably entitled to a good dinner once a week for helping you to develop your "habit."

END NOTES

Metter EJ, Conwit R, Tobin J, Fozard JL' 'Age-associated loss of power and strength in the upper extremities in women and men.'' J Gerontol A Biol Sci Med Sci. Sept.1997 Sep; pp 267-276

CHAPTER 14
FLEXIBILITY AND
COORDINATION

Flexibility results when a person stretches connective tissue: ligaments (which hold bone to bone); tendons (which hold muscle to bone); fascia (a sheet of connective tissue); and small pieces of connective tissue that hold the muscle fibers together. On the muscle chart the connective tissue appears in white.

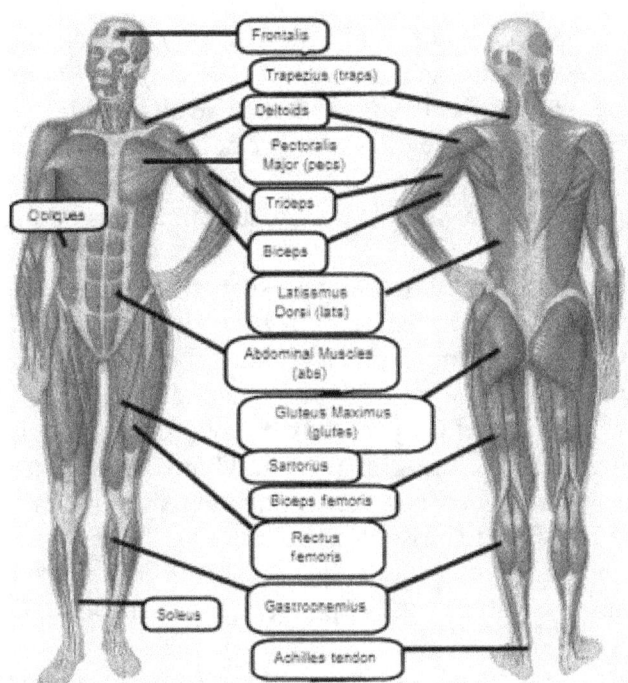

Connective tissue shrinks somewhat if it is not stretched often. We often feel a tightness in the lower back or a lessened ability to touch our toes as we age. But shrunken or tightened connective tissue can be stretched relatively easily, and normal flexibility can usually be regained within a few weeks time, if the proper stretching exercises are done daily. It is never too late to start. A recent study of women with an average age of 72 showed significant increases in flexibility after a 10 week stretching program. (1We actually need more stretching as we age because of the tightness and the loss of elasticity in our muscle fibers.

One of the chief causes of poor posture is tight connective tissue. When the tissue in the front of the shoulders is allowed to shrink, it pulls the shoulders forward resulting in round shoulders. When the tissue, which connects the lower hips to the thigh, is allowed to shorten, it pulls the hips forward and a "pot belly" develops. Pot belly can also be caused by too much beer, too many cakes, and weak abdominal muscles.

Two flexibility exercises that help to prevent poor posture (or assist in regaining good posture) are the chest stretcher and the lower hip stretcher.

The exercise which best stretches the front of the shoulders is done by pulling the shoulders and arms back as far as they can go in a slow stretch. This not only stretches the front of the shoulder area but also strengthens the upper back which will aid in helping to pull the shoulders back.

The exercise that best stretches the front of the lower hip area is done by taking a normal stride forward, tightening the abdominal muscles (so that they will not be

151

stretched) then pushing the hips forward until the stretch is felt in the front of the lower hips.

Three exercises for general flexibility should also be done. The best exercise for trunk flexibility is done by twisting the body as far as it will go. Push with the shoulder to accentuate the twisting action. The stretch is very good for the lower back and may be felt in the knees or ankles, if done correctly.

The best exercise for stretching the lower back and the back of the thighs is done in a sitting position. Reach toward the toes as far as possible. This exercise is more effective when sitting than when standing because the back of the thighs are relaxed when sitting. When standing they are under tension.

Stretching the calf muscle (back of the lower leg) is done by standing a few feet from a wall, placing the hands on the wall, and with the feet flat on the floor lean forward from the ankles until you feel the stretch in the calf muscle and heel cord (Achilles tendon). Women who have worn high heel shoes generally have allowed the Achilles tendon to shorten more than normal so will need additional stretching.

The American College of Sports Medicine suggests that adults should:

Do flexibility exercises at least two or three days each week to improve their range of motion.

Each stretch should be held for 10-30 seconds to the point of tightness or slight discomfort.

Repeat each stretch two to four times, accumulating 60 seconds per stretch.

(static, dynamic, ballistic and PNF stretches are all effective.)

Warm up because flexibility exercise is most effective when the muscle is warm. Try light aerobic activity or a hot bath to warm the muscles before stretching.

Good posture requires not only the flexibility to allow the shoulders and hips to be able to assume the proper alignment but also the strength to hold that alignment. The major muscle groups which hold one in a good posture are: the gluteal muscles of the buttocks, which pull down on the back of the hips, in turn raising the front of the hips; the abdominal muscles, which pull up on the front of the hips; the lower back muscles, which pull down on the rib cage, raising the chest; and the upper back muscles which hold the shoulders back.

The best exercise for the abdominal muscles is the curl-up. While sitting on the floor with the knees bent, the trunk is curled forward as far as possible without letting the belt (top of hips) rise from the floor. Keeping the hips on the floor and the knees bent makes it nearly impossible to use the muscles in the lower hip area These are the muscles which tend to pull the hips forward, giving one a pot belly and a sway back. Put your hands on your chest, look up at the ceiling, and curl forward. This exercise should be done ten to 50 times each day. If you can't do the exercise, grab the back of your thighs with your hands and pull yourself up. In this way your biceps will aid you in doing the curl up.

If you are not sufficiently strong to perform the abdominal curl up, there is a progression of exercises that can be done to strengthen the muscles. Lie on the floor. If you are very weak, bend one leg then lift it towards your shoulders. (Very few people are sufficiently weak to have to start with this exercise.) The next level of progression is lifting both legs bent. When you can do this ten times you will be ready for the real curl up--holding the back of the thighs.

The exercise that strengthens all of the back muscles is the back extension. Raise the shoulders and legs upward 2 to 4 inches, then relax. This should also be done ten to 50 times. This may be the most important exercise one can do, since the lower back muscles are the most often injured. It therefore behooves us to keep them as strong as possible to minimize the chance of injury. Lower back pain afflicts nearly 7 million people. It is often a result of poor posture, but can be caused by muscle weakness, muscle strain, mental stress, poor sleeping habits, and other causes.

Think tall for better posture. Stand tall, walk tall, sit tall. When you stretch to be as tall as possible, all of the right things happen. The abdominal and lower back muscles tighten. The chest is raised while the abdomen is flattened. However, if your shoulders are rounded or your head is held forward, "standing tall" will not change these. However, when you stand tall, the shoulders are rotated backward so that gravity and the large chest muscles do not exert as much forward pull on them. This makes it easier to hold them back.

There is probably no better way to feel like we did when we were younger than to carry ourselves with a good posture.

NEUROMUSCULAR COORDINATION

As we age many of our physical abilities are likely to reduce. Coordination and balance are commonly affected. Often it is an aging of a part of the brain, such as the cerebellum. Sometimes it is a result of nerve damage from surgeries such as hip or knee replacements or from injuries sustained when we were younger. Often it is merely because we have stopped doing physical activities that require physical coordination—other than changing TV channels with a remote control!

The American College of Sport Medicine suggest that:

We do exercises for coordination and balance two or three days per week.

Exercises should involve motor skills (balance, agility, coordination and gait--proprioceptive exercise training and multifaceted activities (tai ji and yoga) to improve physical function and prevent falls in older adults.

20-30 minutes per day is appropriate for neuromotor exercise.

AND MORE

The ACSM also warns that pedometers should not be used as the only measurement of activity. While it may show some activity in terms of aerobic endurance, they do not indicate strength workouts or neuromuscular exercise. Additionally, we must be concerned that we sit too much – – even if we are getting the minimum amount of recommended activities. So we also need to keep track of our sedentary time. Sitting at the office, sitting reading, watching television and other such non-active occupations can be seen as negative in terms of our over all lifestyle.(2)

WHAT YOU CAN DO FOR YOURSELF

Balance tends to reduce as we get older. Balance is a combination of the coordination of nerves in the brain (especially the cerebellum); the ability of your eyes to tell your brain when you are wavering; and the nerves in your legs. If you have had the surgery, such as knee or hip replacement, nerves may have been damaged during the surgery. Balance exercises are designed to assist one or more of these coordination factors to function more efficiently.

Exercises for balance (be able to stabilize yourself by having your hands on or near a table, sofa or chair.

Stand on one foot at least 15 seconds. Then on the other foot.

Stand with both feet together and close your eyes.

Stand on your toes and close your eyes.

Walk on your toes.

Extend your hand high and somewhat to the side, move it around and follow it with your eyes.

Turn around to your right and to your left. When you can do it easily with your eyes open, do it with your eyes closed.

Coordination is the ability to move your body in the way you would like. As we get older our coordination often deteriorates.

Exercises for coordination.

Bounce a ball. Bounce it continually, like a basketball dribble.

Bounce a tennis ball and catching one-handed. Bounce a volleyball and capture with two hands.

Throw ball against the wall and catch it.

Hop on one leg.

Skip.

Close your eyes and with your palms straight out to the side, touch your finger to your nose.

Move your tongue as fast as you can up and down, then side to side

END NOTES

Rider, R. A. and Daly, J. "Effects of flexibility training on enhancing spinal mobility in older women." Journal of Sports Medicine and Physical Fitness. 31(2) June 1991, pp. 213-217.

http://www.acsm-msse.org/; see also their main site: www.acsm.org.

CHAPTER 15
CONSIDERATIONS--BEFORE YOU EXERCISE

We will assume that a large number of you will be walking or running for fitness. There are a few things you can do to make your exercise more pleasant and to reduce your chances of any injury.

YOUR SHOES

When you walk into an athletic-shoe store, chances are you'll be overwhelmed by the selection and feel the urge to buy the shoes endorsed by sports celebrities. Superstores may carry hundreds of different joggers from a dozen major manufacturers.. And the same goes for most other types of athletic shoes, from walkers and cross-trainers to basketball shoes and football cleats.

If there is a shoe store with special apparatus, such as treadmills with computerized photo equipment for foot analysis, and trained personnel, you may be able to leave the decisions up to the experts. If you don't have such a podiatric luxury you will need to spend a few minutes getting to know your feet and ankles.

Before you shop you should get to know your feet and analyze how you will use your new shoes—for walking, running, aerobics, squash, or an other sport. Will you be exercising on grass or on concrete? The harder the surface, the greater shock absorbing qualities you will need. Without adequate shock absorbing qualities you may be setting yourself up for shin splints. So runners and high impact aerobics exercisers must think about the quality of the sole.

Just as human feet vary, so do sports and fitness levels. For example, if you only jog a little every week or kick the soccer ball around with your grandchild from time to time, an all-purpose cross-training shoe should be fine. But if you do a certain sport or activity three or more times a week, you should wear shoes specific to that sport or activity; they may help you avoid injuries such as "shin splints" or ankle sprains.

As we age our bodies do deteriorate. We may still think like 25 year olds but our bodies are showing the wear and tear of all of those years of living the good life. Even if we have exercised throughout our lives our bodies will become more susceptible to overuse injuries. We therefore must be much more particular with our shoes, the surface on which we exercise, and any warnings our body gives us relative to pain. (1)

In general, people who run or do aerobics need shoes with a lot of impact-absorbing cushioning. Walkers need stiffer shoes that have extra shock absorption at the heel as well as soles that provide a good roll off the toes. Running shoes are more flexible than walking shoes. People who play court sports need shoes that help keep the ankle stable during side-to-side movements, which means that the sole can't be too thick. So if do several types of fitness activities you may need several different types of shoes.

Which features do you need? To begin with, you should know if your feet have high, medium, or low arches. It's easy to tell which kind you have. Just wet the bottom of your bare foot and make a footprint on a hard surface. If the forefoot and heel areas are connected by a mark about an inch wide, you have high-arched feet. If the footprint looks somewhat like the shape of your foot, you have a low arch. A medium arch falls somewhere in between.

For a foot with a high arch, a less flexible foot, you will want a more cushioned sole. If you are flat-footed, your feet are probably too flexible, and you would want a stiffer shoe. Those who have medium arches would want something in the middle—a so-called "stability shoe."

Keep in mind any foot problems you've had and try to find a shoe that can accommodate them. Do you have a history of ankle sprains? Then perhaps you should have a high-topped shoe for better ankle support. Have you had deep arch pain? Maybe you need a special arch support. Do you have bunions? Then you need a shoe with a wide toe box.

Women should be cautious when selecting shoes. Downsized men's shoes have long been offered as "women's" shoes, and some still are. But their heels can be too loose, which prompts women to wear smaller sizes that can cause problems. Women should seek out shoes that fit their feet properly. Some companies, including Nike, Adidas, and Reebok, now offer models specifically designed for women's feet. Saucony is noted for shoes that fit women's feet well, because its shoes tend to have narrower heels.

Bring your workout socks and your orthotics if you use them. Your new shoes should feel comfortable right a way.

Monitor the condition of your shoes as they get older. After about 400 or 500 miles (300 to 700 miles depending on the shoe and our own weight), the cushioning on most shoes wears out. However some of the air cell shoes and gel cushions may last longer.

Ankle braces. If your ankles are prone to sprains it is a good idea to wear ankle braces. This is particularly true when playing court and field games and running on an uneven surface, but even running on a flat surface may create problems—especially if you are running on a sidewalk and must go up and down curbs occasionally. Ankle braces can encircle the ankle with a rather stiff cloth which is held tight with laces or Velcro or they can be open stabilizers with plastic or metal sides. These give the ankle more up and down flexibility but still stop the sideways movement which causes the sprain. They cost about twice as much as the simpler braces. (about $30)

An ankle brace that reduces the overpronation of the ankle and foot may assist in preventing overuse injuries. (2)

Sport surfaces are also more important as we age. Sand or grass are much more forgiving than asphalt or concrete. They should therefore be much easier on our aging joints. Another medium is water. You can swim or run in the pool or lake. Running in water, called deep water running, is done with a weight supporting life vest. It is found to be even more strenuous than running on the ground and it doesn't have any negative effects on our bones or joints. (3)

USING THE RIGHT CLOTHING

You will naturally dress depending on two factors, the weather and your activity. For example if you are a cross country skier you may be out for 4 to 6 hours. You will be working hard but you don't really want to sweat. Consequently you will dress in a number of layers. As you warm up you will remove successive layers so that the cold air will neutralize your body's heat.

On cold days be certain to dress warm. More layers are better than one or two layers because each layer traps air which is an insulator. It is essential to keep your muscles warm so that they can perform efficiently and not cramp. You will want to avoid the possibility of frostbite or other cold weather problems. Keep your ears, nose, fingers and toes warm.

If you are a skier or a mountain climber always keep a mask, hat and gloves handy. And be certain that you have warm socks. A friend recently lost several of his toes to frostbite while climbing in Chile during the winter.

If you are running on a hot day you will want to wear as little as possible so that the perspiration on your skin will be evaporated quickly and cool you down. Excess heat not only negatively affects your performance and comfort, but it also can be a source of serious health problems such as heat exhaustion and sun stroke.

As the outside temperature increases it becomes less and less possible to get rid of the heat of the body which exercise produces. For example, if exercising at 3 degrees C (37 F) you are 20% more effective in eliminating body heat than if you are exercising at 20 degrees C (78 F) and 150% more effective than if you were exercising at 40 degrees C

(104 F). It is not uncommon for the body to reach a temperature of 40 to 41 degrees C (104 to 105 F) when exercising. But normal resting body temperature is 37 degrees C (98.6 F). The high heat makes it difficult, or impossible, for the perspiration to evaporate so the body can't be effectively cooled.

The heat generated in the muscles is released by:

--Conduction--from the warmer muscles to the cooler skin;

--Convection--of the heat loss from the skin to the air; and

--Evaporation--of the perspiration being vaporized.

Conduction occurs through the body's liquids, such as the blood, absorbing the heat created by the contraction of the muscles and moving it to the cooler skin. Water can absorb many thousands of times more heat than can air, so blood is an excellent conductor of heat from the muscles.

Convection occurs when the heat near the skin is absorbed into the atmosphere. For a swimmer in a cool pool, effective convection is very easy. For the runner it is more difficult. It is aided by a lower air temperature and by wind.

Wind affects the body temperature by cooling it faster than the registered temperature would warrant. We have all heard of the wind chill factor present on colder days. The wind makes the body experience more cold than would be expected by the actual temperature. (See chart.) But even on warmer days the wind will evaporate the perspiration and cool the body faster than might otherwise be expected. This may increase the need for fluids to continue the production of sweat. A four mile an hour wind is twice as effective in cooling as is a one mile an hour wind. (This is the basis for the Wind Chill Factor associated with winds in cool environments.)

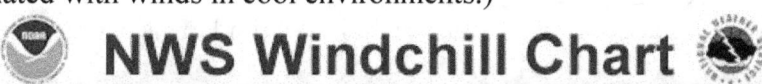

NWS Windchill Chart

Calm	for Temperature (°F)																	
	40	35	30	25	20	15	10	5	0	-5	-10	-15	-20	-25	-30	-35	-40	-45
5	36	31	25	19	13	7	1	-5	-11	-16	-22	-28	-34	-40	-46	-52	-57	-63
10	34	27	21	15	9	3	-4	-10	-16	-22	-28	-35	-41	-47	-53	-59	-66	-72
15	32	25	19	13	6	0	-7	-13	-19	-26	-32	-39	-45	-51	-58	-64	-71	-77
20	30	24	17	11	4	-2	-9	-15	-22	-29	-35	-42	-48	-55	-61	-68	-74	-81
25	29	23	16	9	3	-4	-11	-17	-24	-31	-37	-44	-51	-58	-64	-71	-78	-84
30	28	22	15	8	1	-5	-12	-19	-26	-33	-39	-46	-53	-60	-67	-73	-80	-87
35	28	21	14	7	0	-7	-14	-21	-27	-34	-41	-48	-55	-62	-69	-76	-82	-89
40	27	20	13	6	-1	-8	-15	-22	-29	-36	-43	-50	-57	-64	-71	-78	-84	-91
45	26	19	12	5	-2	-9	-16	-23	-30	-37	-44	-51	-58	-65	-72	-79	-86	-93
50	26	19	12	4	-3	-10	-17	-24	-31	-38	-45	-52	-60	-67	-74	-81	-88	-95
55	25	18	11	4	-3	-11	-18	-25	-32	-39	-46	-54	-61	-68	-75	-82	-89	-97
60	25	17	10	3	-4	-11	-19	-26	-33	-40	-48	-55	-62	-69	-76	-84	-91	-98

Wind (mph)

Frostbite Times ■ 30 minutes ■ 10 minutes □ 5 minutes

$$\text{Wind Chill (°F)} = 35.74 + 0.6215T - 35.75(V^{0.16}) + 0.4275T(V^{0.16})$$

Where, T= Air Temperature (°F)   V= Wind Speed (mph)   *Effective 11/01/01*

Evaporation is the most effective method for cooling the body which is exercising in the air. Each liter of sweat which evaporates takes with it 580 kilocalories. This is enough heat to raise the temperature of ten liters of water 58 degrees Celsius (ten and a half quarts of water 105 degrees F). As the skin is cooled by the evaporation of the sweat, the skin is able to take more of the heat from the blood and thereby cool the blood so that it can pick up more heat from the muscles. For this reason it is not recommended to change to dry clothes when you are sweating on a hot day. As more perspiration is evaporated from your wet clothes you will get a greater cooling effect.

Humidity is the most important factor regulating the evaporation of one's sweat.

High humidity reduces the ability of the perspiration to be evaporated. It is the evaporation of the sweat which produces the cooling effect as the perspiration goes from liquid to gas. Exercising in a rubber suit has similar effects to exercising in high humidity because the water cannot evaporate. Rubber suits are therefore not recommended.

REPLACING YOUR FLUIDS

The ingredients of sweat change as you exercise. At the beginning there are a number of salts excreted. Sodium chloride (common table salt) as well as potassium, calcium, chromium, zinc, and magnesium salts can be lost. The initial sweat contains most of these salts but as the exercise continues, the amount of salts in the sweat is reduced because some of the body's hormones come into play. Aldosterone, for example, conserves the sodium for the body. Consequently the longer we exercise the more that our sweat resembles pure water.

A normal diet replaces all of the necessary elements lost in sweat. Drinking a single glass of orange or tomato juice replaces all or most of the calcium, potassium and magnesium lost. Further, most of us have plenty of sodium in our daily diets.

While there are "fluid replacement" drinks on the market, they are usually not recommended. Water, the most needed element, is slowed in its absorption if it contains other elements such as these salts and sugar. Water alone is therefore the recommended drink for fluid replacement. For those who want to replace water and sugars for energy, the best drinks are those which contain glucose polymers (maltodextrins). So if you are using fluid replacement drinks, check the label. Both caffeine (coffee, tea, and cola drinks) and alcohol dehydrate the body so should be avoided.

Adequate fluid is essential to the functioning of an efficient body. When body fluids are reduced by sweating less fluid is available in the blood and other tissues. These make the body less efficient and, in some cases, can result in serious sickness or even death. To keep the body hydrated you should have frequent breaks for fluid intake. However, even frequent breaks seldom give you enough fluid. The thirst does not signal the true need for fluids. It is therefore better to plan sufficient breaks and drink more water than you think you need.

Dehydration due to excessive heat and/or inadequate fluid intake can cause serious heat related illnesses. A sudden change in the heat or humidity, such as occurs when you train or travel to a warmer or more humid climate, to compete can cause problems. If you were to travel to India, Egypt or the Caribbean to compete in a marathon or a soccer match it would probably take 10 days to two weeks to acclimatize yourself to the warmer or more humid climate.

A tennis player may lose 1/2 to 2 1/2 liters of water in an hour. Older athletes, women, and those not accustomed to exercising in heat have the biggest problems. As much as 1 1/2 liters of water may be lost before one feels thirsty. It is therefore essential to keep drinking water or other fluid replacement drinks. (4)

Among the changes that will probably occur are: a reduced heart rate (due to less need for blood to heat the skin resulting in less blood flow to the skin), an increase in the amount of blood plasma, increased sweating, perspiring earlier when exercising, increased salt losses, and the psychological adjustments made to the experiencing greater heat and humidity.

A comprehensive French study of blood changes during a marathon has indicated that the sodium ions were not significantly reduced and potassium actually increased. This may make us question the need for these in sports drinks. However the sugars and water in the sports drinks may be needed. The average marathon runner loses about 4 pounds during the race. Most of this is water with some of it coming from the use of sugars (glycogen) and body fats. (About 2900 kilocalories are used in a marathon run.) During the run the body creates some water as it uses the glycogen. About 36 ounces is produced in this process. Urination is also decreased thereby saving the body's water store. (5)

SKIN PROBLEMS

People who exercise are prone to numerous skin problems caused by increased moisture (athlete's foot), friction (blisters) or damaging elements like cold, sunlight, and infection. Most skin problems, however, can be prevented by keeping the skin dry, clean, and protected.

Sweating is a common cause of skin problems. Wet skin promotes the proliferation of otherwise normal skin bacteria and other microscopic organisms. Foot odor, for example, is largely due to bacteria that thrive in a moist environment. These same bacteria can also cause pitted keratolysis, a foul-smelling condition in which tiny pits appear on the heels and soles.

Jock itch (tinea cruris) and athlete's foot (tinea pedis) also occur more often in moist conditions. Continuing to wear wet clothing after a workout also increases the risk of folliculitis, a bacterial infection of the hair follicles. Infections like impetigo and bacterial folliculitis can also spread via surfaces like padded workout benches and the handles on weight machines. Warm, moist conditions allow these organisms to thrive. Preventing ''jock itch'' requires that you keep the skin of the groin as dry as possible. Loose pants and underwear allow more air to reach these areas. Exercisers should bathe and change clothes (including underwear) as soon as possible after working out Antibacterial soap can also help keep the bacteria count down.. Thorough drying of the skin is also important.

Socks should be absorbent or made of synthetic material that "wicks" away moisture. Go barefoot or wear sandals when possible to allow your feet to be moisture free. Your shoes should be allowed to dry for at least 24 hours between uses. Feet should be washed and rinsed well every day, and then thoroughly dried. (A hair dryer may help.) In addition, benzoyl peroxide 5% or 10% gel or a spray underarm antiperspirant that contains aluminum chlorhydrate or aluminum chloride can be applied to the feet once or twice daily.

People who have repeated bouts of athlete's foot can apply over-the-counter antifungal products such as miconazole nitrate, tolnaftate, or clotrimazole to help prevent reoccurances.

Friction is another common cause of skin problems. Chafing often occurs in areas where skin rubs clothing or another skin surface. Blisters typically appear in thicker, pressure-bearing areas such as the palms of the hands and the soles of the feet. Friction from clothing can also cause an irritation, and even bleeding, of the nipples, often called jogger's nipples. Improper shoes or socks can aid in the development of blisters on the back of the heel. Petroleum jelly applied to areas prone to rubbing or chafing can also help--not only for chafing, but for blisters and jogger's nipples as well. Soft, light, smooth fabric should be worn to avoid jogger's nipples. Bras decrease friction, which probably explains why men have jogger's nipples more than women do. Also, adhesive bandages can be placed over nipples to reduce friction.

Blisters occur most commonly on the feet from rubbing between skin and footwear. Shoes should fit well and be gradually broken in before using them in athletic activities. Use the same drying measures described for athlete's foot, because moisture increases friction between skin and fabric. Wearing a thin pair of socks under thicker, more absorbent socks can also decrease friction.

Cold and sun exposure can cause skin problems or aggravate existing conditions. Common weather-related problems include frostbite, dry skin, sunburn, and fever blisters.

Those prone to fever blisters should apply a sunscreen-containing lip balm before going outdoors and then reapply it frequently. Very susceptible people may wish to consult their doctor about preventive drugs like acyclovir.

In most situations, sunburn is easily avoided with the use of protective clothing and sunscreen. Hats and clothing made of tightly woven fabric provide fairly good protection against the sun's harmful ultraviolet rays. Caps protect the scalp and, to some degree, the face. Broad-brimmed hats afford additional coverage of the ears. Waterproof sunscreens with a sun protection factor (SPF) of at least 15 should be applied to exposed skin 20 to 30 minutes before going out in the sun.

To prevent frostbite, wear layers of non-restricting clothing in cold weather, paying special attention to the ears, cheeks, nose, fingers, and toes. Check yourself regularly for areas of extreme cold or numbness--especially if you have pain that suddenly stops. Also, check your companions' faces and ears frequently for loss of color or other signs of freezing. Any area of suspected frostbite should be warmed as soon as possible, but do not rub or massage the skin because rubbing may worsen any damage.

Winter dry skin can be minimized by moisturizing the skin. Bathing and showering should be brief and as cool as tolerable, since prolonged exposure to hot water depletes natural skin oils. Use mild "moisturizing" soaps. After bathing, the skin should be patted, not rubbed, with a towel. Apply moisturizing lotion or cream immediately after bathing and any time the skin feels dry, especially before going outdoors. Direct contact with wool should be avoided because it can irritate dry skin.

OTHER INJURIES

Women are more likely than men to ankle and knee sprains, stress fractures, shin splints, and hip problems when running or playing sports which involve running. Men are more likely to suffer injuries to the front of the thigh (quadriceps), plantar fascitis (pain under the foot), or Achilles tendon problems. (6)

Wearing effective braces (such as ankle braces or tennis elbow braces) can reduce your chance of injury. Running on softer surfaces, doing low impact aerobics, or doing "deep water running" can also greatly reduce stress and impact type injuries.

END NOTES

Ting, A. "Running and the older athlete." Clinics in Sports Medicine. 10(2) Apr. 1991. Pp. 319-325.

LeClercq, D. "Ankle bracing in running: the effect of a push type medium ankle brace upon movements of the foot and ankle during the stance phase," International Journal of Sports Medicine. 18(3) Apr. 1997. Pp. 222-228.

Swedenhag, J. and Seger, J. "Running on land or in water: comparative exercise physiology" Medicine and Science in sports and Exercise. 24(10) Oct. 1992, pp. 1155-1160.

Bergeron, M. et al "Fluid and Electrolyte losses during tennis in the heat" Racquet Sports: Clinics in Sports Medicine. Vol 14:1Jan. 1995. W.B.Saunders, Philadelphia, 1995, p. 23.

Pastene, J. et al. "Water balance during and after marathon running." European Journal of Applied Physiology, 73 (1 and 2) 1996, pp. 49-55

See: O'Connor, B. et al. Sports Injuries and Illnesses. Crowood Press. 1998. This book will give you the symptoms, treatment and prevention strategies for most sports related injuries.)

CHAPTER 16
UNDERSTANDING OUR STRESSES

We all encounter stresses. They may be life threatening or merely inconveniences. How we handle them can be the difference between being mentally healthy and mentally ill. Life is a forceful teacher. It has a persistent method of presenting the same lesson again and again until we learn it. But we want to learn it as simply as possible!

Handling stresses throughout our lives helps us to age positively. As we age the stresses of our earlier live, such as getting good grades in school or getting another job promotion give way to the stresses that are appropriate to our age. Our parents and friends fall ill or die. Our children struggle financially or psychologically with divorce or drugs. Our retirement benefits don't go as far as we had hoped because of inflation. Every age has its stresses. Every stress can be confronted—but not always conquered to our satisfaction. Wrinkles come and hair goes. How do we handle the challenges of our age?

Stress can be said to be the response which the mind and body make when psychological requirements are too high. (1) For example writing a letter firing an employee and writing a letter to a friend, both experiences in writing, will probably cause different levels of stress. Stress can also be a physical condition, such as the effect of excess cold or heat on the body.

It is not the cause of the stress, as much as the effect of that stress on the individual, which is the major concern. Loud rock music may be pleasant for one person and a terrible noise to another. Giving a speech before an unknown group of people can be either stimulating or unpleasant depending on the situation.

Individuals who think well of themselves may experience less stress. Their positive feelings make them less likely to be overcome by the stressor and they are more likely to feel in control-rather than have the stressor in control. Studies on humans, at the International Centre for Health and Society at University College in London, and studies on baboons, in Kenya's Serengeti, strongly indicate that the higher an individual is in the hierarchy of the society or of one's job classification, the longer the individual lived. It seems that both a lower class baboon or a lower class human had less control over their lives and therefore had more life stress. This was true for humans even when other risk factors were controlled such as smoking, cholesterol level, and blood pressure. So self esteem and the ability to control one's life are certainly positive factors and stress reducers. (2) Many studies have shown the effects of stress, including the lack of control of one's behavior at work, to increased stress and its resulting illness. This does not seem to be a recent occurrence. References to 19th century England's medical schools and the dissection of cadavers showed that the cadavers from lower social class people had much larger adrenal glands than did their higher social class compatriots. This overworking of the adrenal glands can be directly related to their stress. (3)

The effects of unhealthy stress on the person

"Recent literature has emphasized the potential importance of psychosocial stress. Chronic stress is expected to increase the risk of premature death directly through the immune and neuroendocrine systems and indirectly through adverse behavioral responses such as smoking, excessive drinking, and violence behavioral responses to chronic stress may vary from country to country, as is suggested by variations between countries in national patterns of causes of death. Similarly, exposure to chronic stress in disadvantaged groups may increase their risk of different causes of death in different parts of Europe." (4)

The mind and body can react to stressors with anxiety, depression, or hostility. (5) These mental reactions can then be transformed into physical diseases such as heart attack, high blood pressure, ulcers, neck and back pains, and asthma. Now we find that even cancers and other illnesses are related to a lowering of the immune system--which is a possible result of stress. The role of stress in the causing of mental diseases has been known longer but its biochemical effects are being more effectively studied today. (6) As we age the effects of stresses seem to multiply. A stress at age 20 experienced at age 50 can result in much greater physical changes. Consequently we need to be increasingly aware of stressful factors in our lives as we age and eliminate them or effectively cope with them.

A number of years ago the Holmes-Rahe scale was developed. It took into consideration a number of life events, both positive and negative, and correlated them with diseases. The more events a person experienced during a year the more likely it was that diseases would develop. How do you rate?

Life Events-Life Changes Units
Death of spouse-100-
Divorce-73-
Martial separation-65-
Jail term-63-
Death of close family member-63-
Personal injury or illness-53-
Marriage-50-
Fired at work-47-
Marital reconciliation-45-
Retirement-45-
Change in health of a family member-44-
Pregnancy-40-
Sex Difficulties-39-
Gain of new family member-39-
Business readjustment-39-
Change in financial state-38-
Death of close friend-37-
Change to different line of work-36-
Change in number of arguments with spouse-35-
Mortgage over $100,000 -31-
Foreclosure of mortgage or loan-30-
Change in responsibilities at work-29-

Life Events-Life Changes Units
Son or daughter leaving home-29-
Trouble with in-laws-29-
Outstanding personal achievement-28-
Wife begins or stops work-26-
Begin or end school-26-
Change in living conditions-25-
Revision in personal habits-24-
Trouble with boss-23-
Change in work hours or conditions-20-
Change in residence-20-
Change in schools-20-
Change in recreation-19-
Change in church activities-19-
Change in social activities-18-
Mortgage or loan less than $30,000-17-
Change in sleeping habits-16-
Change in number of family get-togethers-15-
Change in eating habits-15-
Vacation-13-
Christmas alone-12-
Minor violations of the law-11-

Heart attacks during middle age are ten times more common among men than women. We have evidence to believe that this is caused at least in part by women's hormones. This is probably one factor. But Dr. Paul Mills, a psycho-biologist at the University of California at San Diego has found another significant factor. In measuring two neurotransmitters, epinephrine and norepinephrine, both of which are significant in the sympathetic nervous system, men had twice the amounts that women had. This would mean that high blood pressure and other negative stress related body reactions could be twice as high in men when experiencing the same stresses as a woman

Another difference in the effect of stresses between men and women may be in the causes of the stress. Men's levels of stress induced neurotransmitters increased much more during competitive and intellectual challenges. Women's levels increased more dramatically during stressful personal situations. Studies in Europe (Karolinska Institute in Sweden) and in the United States (Cornell Medical Center) indicate that when husbands and wives have the same types of jobs the men's stress levels tend to drop as soon as they leave the office. Women's levels tend to stay high throughout the evening, probably because of the family responsibilities which continue into the evening.

Good Stress and Bad Stress

Dr. Hans Selye, the Canadian researcher who was the pioneer of stress research, tells us that there is good stress (eustress, "eu" from the Greek word for "good") and bad stress (distress). We need stress in our lives but we want to increase the eustress and decrease the distress. We want to have the excitement of playing a tennis match, reading a stimulating novel, or traveling to a new destination. These are eustresses. We want to eliminate or control the distresses--the long drive to work, the hassles with the people at home, the lack of challenge at our jobs.

Stress is natural for humans. If you don't want any stress you should have been a rock. Selye once observed that "Stress is the spice of life." (7) But as we encounter stress we must be able to cope with it, then, if possible, eliminate the negative stresses.

Our intelligence can aid us in understanding the causes of our distresses and some of the methods which can be used to reduce those stresses. Our intelligence can also help us to find the lifestyles, the careers, and the relationships which will yield the greatest amount of eustresses. It is assumed that a "self actualized" life, in which a person experiences a great deal of true joy, will make that person immune to the effects of many negative stresses.

Selye has also captured the importance of stress in our lives when he wrote, "...that man's ultimate aim in life is to express himself as fully as possible, according to his own lights, and to achieve a sense of security. To accomplish this, you must first find your optimal stress level, and then use your adaptation energy at a rate and in a direction adjusted to your innate qualifications and preferences." (8)

The General Adaptation Syndrome (GAS) often occurs when we encounter an unwanted stress. There may be three stages to our adaptation to the stress.

Alarm is the first response. The heart rate increases, the blood pressure rises, the breathing becomes more rapid, and digestion slows. These reactions are caused when the hypothalamus (located in the center of the brain) signals the pituitary (the master gland) to release ACTH (adrenocorticotropic hormone). This hormone stimulates the adrenal glands to release other hormones which activate the sympathetic branch of the autonomic nervous system to release the neurotransmitters epinephrine (adrenaline) and epinephrine. The body is then ready for fight or flight--to attack or withdraw.

This alert and ready state can be elicited by any type of surprise--pleasant or unpleasant. A last second win by your favorite team, an encounter with a mugger, a near accident while driving, or winning the lottery can each start this "excitement" phase of a eustressful or distressful event.

The second stage of the general adaptation syndrome is the calming stage when your body attempts to get itself back to normal. This is called the "resistance stage." The body would like to be in a normal state. This we call "homeostasis." It may take only seconds or minutes to regain homeostasis for a positive or "happy" stress or a minor negative stress. Or it may take a long time to get over the stress. A "post traumatic stress syndrome"* is such a long term negative reaction. This might occur when there is a death of a loved one, the loss of a desired job, or a serious or long term physical injury.

The third stage of adaptation, exhaustion, may occur if the stress continues for a long time. A rat forced to swim to exhaustion repeatedly will eventually give up when put into the water. A person who is daily confronted with heavy stresses, such as a soldier in battle or a policeman in a crime ridden ghetto often succumb to mental exhaustion. This exhaustion can come at the end of a hectic day or after a long period of confronting one or more stresses. Naturally the longer the period a person is under stress, the greater the potential exhaustion.

We may handle stresses by adapting to them, by reducing their effects (coping), or by eliminating them through appropriate thinking and behaviors. If I am a young child and my father continually yells at me I may just accept the fact--adapt to it. If other children in my neighborhood experience the same kind of parental behavior I may assume that it is normal and perhaps the negative effects will be small. Here I would be adapting to the stress.

Both the physical body and the mind can make adaptations to stresses. The body may adjust by a reduced immune function which can result in a lower resistance to diseases and more frequent colds. The person may develop allergies such as asthma, acne, skin rashes. The cardiovascular system may react with higher blood pressure, tightness in the chest, or a more rapidly or stronger beating heart. The blood vessels may react by increasing headaches or by slowing the blood flow to the hands and feet making them feel cold. The muscular system can respond with pains in the back, neck or jaw. The gastrointestinal system can show involvement by diarrhea, constipation, burping, excess gas, or ulcers. The nervous system may show signs such as dizziness, tics, menstrual irregularities, or sleep problems. Psychologically people may react by anger, boredom, depression, hopelessness, irritability, hostility, anxiety, panic, frustration, or fear. The method of adjustment is likely to be inherited, although some people "learn" their adjustments by imitating others.

Perhaps I spend all of my free time watching television or I use alcohol or other drugs to cope with my unhappiness. These of course would be poor adjustments. Or perhaps I work extra hard to gain my boss's approval or I exercise to reduce my tensions These would be more effective and healthier methods of coping with the problem.

There are a number of things that you can do to reduce the effects of the stressors or to eliminate them. Many of the positive things that you can do are the same activities which help you to health in every area of your life--physical fitness, an effective sleep and relaxation regimen, sound nutrition, committed social relationships, a positive attitude toward life, meaningful life goals, and a knowledge of how to change behavior for the better.

Effective adjustments to stress can come about only after we have determined whether or not something can be done about that stress. Assume that a person is in a stressful situation. Suppose that the marriage is unhappy. In such a situation the person should have evaluated the possibilities, looked at the desired goal, then accepted what cannot be changed. Divorce is a possibility. So is marriage counseling. Can this be effectively brought up to the spouse? What if neither person wants to change? The option may then be separation or divorce.

The Chinese character for "crisis" is composed of two words, one means "danger," the other means "opportunity." Perhaps this should be our challenge. Or will that create more stress?

Oftentimes we are faced with stress situations to which we must adjust by non-action. A policeman gives me a traffic ticket. My boss fires me. My party lost the election.

Quite often we can take affirmative action to effectively lessen the stress. I might ask for a transfer to another department if there is a personality conflict with a supervisor. I can go to court to fight the traffic ticket. I can work for my political party so that we can win the next election.

Exercise is often overlooked as an effective method of stress reduction. But when one runs, swims, or hits a tennis ball, there is some stress reduction. We often see only the physiological benefits of exercise without recognizing its mental effects. But it is known that forceful exercise, especially where hitting or kicking is involved, is an efficient way of reducing the effects of stress. Psychologists often use soft foam-filled bats or boxing gloves filled with air as vehicles by which people can take out their frustrations by hitting another person or an inanimate object.

Too often stress is handled by reaching for a tranquilizer, a sleeping pill or an alcoholic beverage. "Boy, I need a drink" is often more of a problem than a solution. Pills and booze are not the effective solutions for which most people hope.

We can control some areas of our lives and reduce stress in other areas. Before we can choose the best method of adjusting to a stress we should:

(1) Look for the causes of the stress. Is it something that can be changed or is it something that must be tolerated? Is it a person or a situation? Or is it possible that the problem is me? Do other people react similarly to what I think is the cause of the problem?

(2) It is not necessary to "win" every confrontation. So evaluate your values and goals. Which ones are unimportant? Which are essential? Must I tolerate some stresses in order to accomplish my greater goal?

(3) Be positive. Too often people concentrate on the negative aspects of a situation. The skunk who said, "I think of my stripe as a racing stripe, " was looking at the positive side of his situation. We often look at our liabilities rather than our assets, our failures rather than our successes. Successful adjustments require a positive approach to do something about the stressful situation.

(4) Seek advice. A friend or a professional counselor may be able to give new insights, and certainly will be able to relieve tensions. Talking over a problem is, itself, a tension reliever.

(5) Do one thing at a time. The seconds pass in single file, but they quickly become minutes, hours, . . . and years. When we concentrate on one thing at a time we will be more likely to be able to solve the stressful situation in a rational manner. We will be more likely to find a satisfying solution.

(6) Keep in mind that while each of us has similarities, each of us is unique. Others' problems are not necessarily exactly like our own. But since similarities exist, we may find some possible solutions to our stress problems by reading what others have done in like situations or by attending a type of group therapy such as Alcoholics Anonymous, Gamblers Anonymous, Overeaters Anonymous, or those groups led by professionals.

(7) Train ourselves to recognize an impending personal crisis. Emotional upsets at work, arguments in our marriages, and break-ups with people with whom we feel close, can initiate a mental problem.

If we are "up tight," anxiety-producing situations should be avoided. Societal problems on TV, violent movies or stress-filled family situations can accent our stresses. What we often need is a vacation, a restful outing, or a quiet time, to lessen the feeling of anxiety.

THE IMPORTANCE OF RECOGNIZING OUR STRESSES

The diseases listed earlier are often brought on by uncontrolled stresses. An unhappy marriage or job situation grates on us and affects our immune systems. Not only are we unhappy but we are shortening our lives. When we are not happy we must not accept our fate but we must look for the cause or causes of the problem. Then we must look to see whether we can eliminate the problem, adjust to it, or reduce the consequences of the stress placed on our lives.

AND MORE

SELF TEST 1 What are the major stresses in my life?

Rate 1 to 5 (with 1 meaning "little or no problem" and 5 being "the most severe and bothersome")

1. I don't have enough time to do what I need to do._____
2. Deadlines for jobs at work are problems.___
3. My friends and family make too many demands on my time.___
4. I have at least one boss who bothers me a lot._____
My economy is not in good shape—I need more money._____
I don't have time for recreation. _____
7. I don't know what I want to do with my life._____

8. I am having trouble with my relationship (or finding a relationship).____
9. I worry about my children.____
10. (Other problem[s])_____ bothers me a great deal.____
According to this evaluation the three major stresses in my life are:
1
2.
3.

Self Test 2 (Stress symptoms)
Rate 1 to 5 (1 being the least amount of problem)
1. I put off doing important things (procrastination)____
2. I can't slow down my mind.____
3. I don't sleep well (insomnia)____
4. My moods change often.____
5. I always have to be doing something.____
6. I am tired often.____
7. I get impatient often.____
8. I avoid others as often as possible or I am very shy.____
9. I am often angry.____
10. I am often very sad.____
Which three adjustments do you make the most often?
1._____
2._____
3._____

SELF TEST 3 (Being under control)
(Developed by Aerobics Research, Dallas, TX. Published by Reebok.--by permission)
Answer the YES or NO question then rate the level at which you could manage the stress:
0 10 20 30 40 ` 50 60 70 80 90 100
Very uncertain Somewhat certain Very certain

1. You are trying to concentrate, but you are constantly being interrupted. YES NO _____

2. You must perform a very boring task. YES NO _____
3. You have been thinking about someone who hurt you in the past. YES NO _____

4. You have a neighbor who plays loud music all the time YES NO _____
5. You have several things to finish in a very short time. YES NO _____
6. You are home by yourself and feel lonely. YES NO _____
7. You are in a crowded bus and cannot get to the exit in time for your stop. YES NO _____

8. You keep thinking about an unpleasant experience. YES NO _____
9. You have taken on more than you are able to do. YES NO _____
10. You are waiting by the street for someone to pick you up, and you are getting cold. YES NO _____
11. Although you have plenty of time, you are worried that you will be late for a appointment. YES NO _____
12. Your closest friend left town and you feel alone. YES NO _____
13. You are in a room that is extremely hot. YES NO _____
14. You must buy a gift for someone and the stores are closing.YES NO _____
15. You saw someone being robbed and keep imagining that it could happen to you. YES NO _____
16. You must wait for a delivery and you have nothing to do. YES NO _____

17. Your friends keep asking you to do things you do not have time to do. YES NO
_____

18. You must get a prescription filled, and you can't find a drug store that is open. YES NO _____

19. You have just spent a good deal of time in a place that is very noisy.YES NO
_____

20. Although you have tried your hardest, you have not been able to finish your work. YES NO _____

AND A LITTLE POETRY TO THINK ABOUT
This above all to thine own self be true,
And it must follow, as night the day,
Thou canst not then be false to any man.
 Shakespeare (Hamlet)
THE MAN IN THE GLASS
When you get what you want in your struggle for self,
 And the World makes you King for a day,
Just go to the mirror and look at yourself
And see what that man has to say.

For it's not your father or mother or wife,
Whose judgment upon you must pass;
The fellow whose verdict will really count most
Is the man staring back from the glass.

You may be like Jack Horner and chisel a plum,
And think you're a wonderful guy;
But the man in the glass knows you're only a bum,
If you can't look him straight in the eye.

He's the one to please -don't mind the rest -
For he's with you clear up to the end;
And you've passed your most dangerous, difficult test
If the man in the glass is your friend.

You may fool all the world, down the pathway of years,
And get pats on the back as you pass;
But your only reward will be heartaches and tears,
If you've cheated the man in the glass.
 Author Unknown

WHEN THINGS GO WRONG
When things go wrong, as they sometimes will,
When the road you're trudging seems all up hill,
When the funds are low, and the debts are high,
And you want to smile, but you have to sigh,
When care is pressing you down a bit,
Rest if you must but don't you quit.

Life is queer with its twists and turns,
As everyone of us sometimes learns,
And many a failure turns about,
When he might have won had he stuck it out,
Don't give up though the pace seems slow,

You may succeed with another blow.

Success is failure turned inside out,
The silver tint of the clouds of doubt,
And you never can tell how close you are,
It may be near when it seems so far,
So stick to the fight when you're hardest hit,
It's when things seem worse,
That you must not quit.
Author unknown

Coping with life threatening illness. (Condensed from "Ways to Cope with Life Threatening Illness, by Spiegel, David. Quoted in The Menninger Letter, June 1994, p 4)

1. Look the illness in the eye. Acknowledge the threat of the danger, then pursue the cure while letting it affect your life as little as possible.

2. Coping is enhanced when people with a similar problem deal with it together. Women in support groups for their cancer problems lived longer than those who were not in such groups.

3. Take it seriously but don't let it take you over. Put it in perspective and take the opportunity to clarify your priorities--projects you wanted to accomplish, friends you want to see, etc.

4. Take control of everything you can and let go of the rest.

STRESSORS

Following is an outline of a few possible stressors. Each may cause great distress to some people and none to others.

POSSIBLE STRESSORS

PHYSICAL

A lack of oxygen.
Extreme fatigue or tiredness.
An excess of lead or asbestos in the environment.
Too much heat or cold
A strong wind.
A loud noise, including loud music.
Some chemicals (some acids or alkalis, alcohol)

BIOLOGICAL

An allergic reaction to poison ivy or poison oak.
An upset stomach from the salmonella germ.
Any disease, injury, or disability
Hunger or thirst
Physical problems of aging

MENTAL

A threat or a perceived threat
Lack of satisfaction of a basic drive (power, love, meaning)
Failure at school or work
Mental problems of aging (each age may have its own problems)
Experiencing a loss, such as death or the break-up of a relationship.
Being in a minority group (racial, ethnic, religious, etc.) if you feel discrimination.

VALUES

Doing something counter to what one's religion holds dear:
---having an abortion when it is considered wrong
---Lying
---Cheating on a test
Doing something counter to another type of value:
--Ordering a second helping when on a diet

--Buying a coat which isn't needed when you are on a tight budget.
SOCIAL RELATIONSHIPS
Not having a good friend.
Unhappiness with parents or children (such as alcoholism or drug use)
ECONOMICS
Not having enough money
Having to pay taxes which are too high.
CAREER
Unhappiness with one's career
Inability to obtain a job
Job pressures
Lack of control and authority on the job
POLITICAL
War or the threat of war.
Injustices carried on by your government or another government
Being involved in a law suit
GEOGRAPHICAL
Living in a big city
Living in a ghetto
Living in a third world country
Living in an area which is negatively prejudiced against you
because of your sex, race, or religion.
Living in a country which is very hot, very cold, or has long dark winters.

Work can often be a stress reliever--if it allows us to:
--Get esteem from others,
--Experience real achievement,
--is meaningful,
--uses our knowledge and abilities.
NEGATIVE METHODS OF THINKING
1. All or nothing. Everything is black or white, no gray. Seldom is anything totally good or totally bad. Some people only see the negatives.
2. Overgeneralization. Taking one situation and applying it to all similar situations. "I didn't get that Job. I'll never get a job."
3. Discounting what you have done that is good.
4. Blowing things out of proportion, making them larger or smaller than they are in reality.
5. Mistaking emotional feelings for rational thinking.
6. Jumping to conclusions without all of the evidence being in.
7. Assuming that people are thinking or doing things which will affect you, even though you have no evidence.
8. Labeling yourself as a loser, one who can't get things done.
9. Placing too much guilt on yourself or on others. Get a realistic share of the blame based on the evidence.

--Things to do today--
1) Get up
2) Survive
3) Go to bed.

READING LIST OF SOME CLASSICS IN STRESS REDUCTION
Benson, Herbert. Your Maximum Mind. New York: Times Books. 1987.
Bolles, Richard. What Color is Your Parachute? A practical manual for job-hunters and career changers. Berkeley, CA: Ten Speed Press. 1994

Friedman, Meyer, and Rosenman, Ray. Type A Behavior and Your Heart. Greenwich, CT: Knopf. 1974

Kabat-Zinn, Jon. Full Catastrophe Living. New York: Delacorte Press. 1990

Needleman, Jacob. Money and the Meaning of Life. New York: Doubleday/Currency. 1991.

Selye, Hans. Stress Without Distress. New York: Lippincott. 1974.

Selye, Hans. Stress in Health and Disease. Reading, MA: Butterworths. 1976.

END NOTES

Don Frankl. Paper delivered to the American Academy of Kinesiology, Washington, D.C. April 1993.

2.Williams S. et al. "Senior house officers' work related stressors, psychological distress, and confidence in performing clinical tasks in accident and emergency: a questionaire study" Brit. Med. Jour. March 1997, 314:7082; and, "Why workers suffer most from stress." Financial Times (London) Feb. 26, 1995, see also Healthy People 2000, p. 60)

Brunner, E. "Socioeconomic determinants of health: Stress and the biology of inequality." Brit Med Jour. May, 1997, 314, p. 1472

4. Kunst, A. et al. "Occupational class and cause specific mortality in middle aged men in 11 European countries: comparison of population based studies." Brit. Med. Jour. 316 p. 7145.

5. Repetti, R.L. "Short term effects of occupational stressors on daily mood and health complaints" Health Psychology, vol. 112, 1993, pp 125-131.

6. Herbert, J. "Stress, the brain, and mental illness." Brit. Med. Jour. Aug. 1997. 315 p.7107.

7. Stress Without Distress. New York: Signet. 1975. p.83.

8. Selye, ibid. p 110.

CHAPTER 17
HANDLING OUR STRESSES

As mentioned, as we age stresses can affect us more severely because our youthful bodies could deal with them more effectively. Consequently we must take stress, or the threat of stress, more seriously as we age. While the ideal way to handle unwanted stresses is to eliminate them, this is not always possible. Consequently we must often learn to handle the stresses with coping skills. These skills can be seen as: relaxation techniques, such as meditation; exercise techniques, such as aerobic dance or swimming; or diversion techniques, such as music or reading.

Coping techniques, which may reduce the effects that distresses have on us, can be:

1) cognitive (from the mind to the body) such as meditation; 2) somatic (from the body to the mind) such as exercise; or 3) behavioral approaches (changing behaviors which are harmful) such as time management. (1)

Cognitive techniques begin with the mind. It is hoped that by correct thinking, or by "non-thinking," the body can be relaxed and the tensions of the ''distresses'' can be reduced. Among the cognitive techniques are meditation, the relaxation response, hypnosis, and thought stopping.

Meditation is a type of ''non-thinking" which the Hindus of India have used for thousands of years. It was one of the methods which they used to unite with the Brahman (the oneness of nature.) During the 1960's the Maharishi Mahesh Yogi came to the the West and both simplified and popularized the idea of meditation. The maharishi taught many people to teach his technique. For a fee a person could be given his or her own private "mantra." That mantra was to be repeated while the person breathed deeply. Using this technique for fifteen to twenty minutes a day once or twice a day proved to be remarkably relaxing. Researchers at Stanford University, along with other institutions, proved that the techniques of the yogi did, in fact, reduce blood pressure and other symptoms of stress. (2) There is a very different set of physiological responses to meditation or the relaxation response than there is to simple rest. (3)

Dr. Herbert Benson, a cardiologist at the Harvard Medical School, acknowledged that Transcendental Meditation can accomplish many of these relaxation techniques, so he wrote a book called, The Relaxation Response (4) He wrote that meditation can be done by almost anyone without special lessons. It doesn't have to be a religious experience.

His directions are to sit in a comfortable chair in a quiet room. Assume a restful position. Close your eyes. Try to relax all your muscles. Then breathe through your nose and become aware of your breathing. Just think about your breathing, and as you breathe out you say to yourself silently some one syllable word which can free the mind from logical thought. You might use the word "one" or "on" or the Hindu word "om" which is often used by Yogis as a mantra. The objective of the word is to take away your normal thoughts. Don't use a word like "sex" or "money"--they will keep your mind active.

Do this breathing, relaxing, and repeating the nonsense word for about 20 minutes. You can open your eyes to check the clock, but it's important that you remain undisturbed for the entire period. Maintain a very passive attitude. Don't worry about how well you are meditating, or you may inhibit the response. If distracting thoughts occur, let them. The meditating word will return naturally.

This relaxation response of Dr. Benson's has been extremely effective in lowering blood pressure. Many relaxation therapists say that anxiety or emotional tension and relaxation are mutually exclusive. You can't be tense if you're relaxed. And it has certainly been proven medically and psychologically that where there is anxiety there is muscle tension. But when muscle tension is relieved, so is the anxiety.

Dr. Benson believes that, if we can't do anything about the stressful lives which so many of us lead, we can at least do something to alleviate the damages of such a life. We can take relaxation breaks. We can do something to relax other than reaching for an artificial aid such as a cigarette, a glass of liquor, or a tranquilizer. We might take naps a couple of times each day, use a meditation technique, or use a type of biofeedback. The effects of relaxing on people with specific medical problems, such as high blood pressure and asthma, have been consistently demonstrated. Once a person can use the relaxation response it is possible to drop the blood pressure ten to twenty points with only a few breaths. So what Dr. Benson had found was that at least one part of meditation was merely the control of the parasympathetic system.

In hypnosis the mind is taught to relax through the power of suggestion. Some people are quite susceptible to such suggestion. Others are not. Hypnosis should only be done by a trained and licensed therapist.

Thought stopping is a technique in which unwanted stress producing thoughts are removed. The individual imagines a situation in which the negative thoughts might occur. (Dealing with a discourteous customer at work would be an example.) A timer is set for about three minutes of this imagining. When the timer indicates that the pre-set time is up, the therapist or the patient, yells "stop." The individual then keeps his or her mind blank for about 30 seconds. If the thoughts return the patient again says "stop."

When the individual has been able to do this with the therapist's help, the process is repeated without the therapist's intervention. The third stage is for the patient to substitute positive and assertive thoughts for the undesired negative thoughts." (I will relax during the examination," or, "I am prepared for this job," are examples.) This method of "thought stopping" is often effective in eliminating obsessive stress producing thinking such as worrying,

Mental imagery or visualization is a technique which is common among athletes but it can be used by anyone. This technique involves imagining yourself doing what you want to do or should do in a certain situation. If you are trying to stop smoking after dinner you may imagine yourself chewing gum or taking a walk after dinner. The imagined action can be influential in having you perform that action after dinner. This technique can be used thinking of yourself from the outside, such as watching yourself in a movie, or imagining yourself doing the action-- from the inside.

For example, if your boss is frequently angry at you with no real reason you may learn to tune him or her out and not react with anger. Just see yourself in that situation. See yourself acting more effectively to reduce the effects of the stressor. If you find that you are shy at social gatherings and would like to be more outgoing, imagine yourself going up to people and starting a conversation. (Most people are just as shy as you are and welcome a chance to talk.) So imagine the different kinds of conversations you can start. Mental imagery is a very simple method of making positive changes to stressors.

Somatic (body to mind) techniques are begun with the body as the focus but the mind relaxes as the body responds to the specific technique. Among the somatic techniques are: yoga, progressive relaxation, diaphragmatic breathing, massage, and physical exercise.

Yoga is an ancient Hindu method of religious salvation. The Hindus had several yogas (paths) to religious experience. Hatha yoga, the method which is discussed here, is the method in which the body is controlled, usually by stretching and deep breathing. The Hindu would use this as the starting point for mind control (meditation). Most people in the West who use yoga use it as a relaxing and physical flexibility activity. In using yoga as a relaxing technique one will gain the ability to stretch tensed muscles and will also get the relaxation advantages of diaphragmatic breathing. There are numerous books and classes which can explain the techniques involved.

Diaphragmatic breathing is simply deep breathing using the diaphragm (the major breathing muscle.) Many people do not use the diaphragm properly. They use the auxiliary breathing muscles of the chest and neck. Deep abdominal or diaphragmatic breathing is a method of relaxation which is a part of many other techniques--meditation, relaxation response, progressive relaxation, yoga, swimming, etc. As such it has some of the same benefits as these other activities. The usefulness of the technique is that it does not require a great deal of practice and it can be done anywhere and at any time.

To learn the technique, if you do not already know how to do it, merely lie on the floor. Uncover the abdominal area so that you can see the skin between the lower part of the ribs and the hips. As you breathe see that your abdomen is rising and falling. If your chest, but not your abdomen, is moving up and down you are not using your diaphragm effectively.

Physical exercise can help a person to relax in several ways. It can be a recreational pursuit, a rhythmic endurance exercise, or a pleasant physically fatiguing experience.

A recreational pursuit, such as a game of tennis or golf, a day of downhill skiing, or an afternoon of aggressive sailing can make a person forget about the problems which have created the stressful feelings in one's life.

A rhythmic activity such as distance swimming, running, walking, rowing or cross country skiing can provide both the diversion of a recreational activity and the rhythmic breathing of a meditation session. But for such an exercise to have stress reducing effects several factors must be present. 1) It should be enjoyable. 2) It should be aerobic and should not be considered to be competitive by the participant. 3) It should be of moderate intensity and last at least 20 minutes. (5)

While people generally report that they feel better after exercise, not all exercise is equally beneficial. In fact some exercise can create stress. A competitive runner or swimmer working to exhaustion so that a peak performance can be achieved in the championship meet is such an example. Similarly recreational swimmers swimming in uncomfortably warm water showed an increase in stress. A golfer or tennis player under pressure to win would be another example.

People who are particularly competitive in life may carry that competitiveness into their recreational pursuits and negate the stress reducing benefits which would have accrued if the exercise had truly been recreational. It is important that if exercise is to be used to reduce stress it musty be pleasant--it must be play. Running may be play for one person but work for another.

Many people have experienced a particularly high level of stress relief after 30 to 50 minutes of aerobic activity. This is often called the "exercise high" and is suspected to be related to the brain's reaction to increased endorphins--brain chemicals similar to opium.

If an exerciser, particularly an aerobic exerciser, has participated in the exercise several times a week for more than a year, the psychological benefits are greater. It has been found that for runners who had run at least 30 miles a week for two years, a single episode of high intensity work on a treadmill greatly reduced the anxiety level of that person and increased the alpha brain waves (the waves present during meditation). But this same level of exercise for people who were not long time runners did not produce these same levels of relaxation. (6) These stress reduction benefits increased as the number of exercise sessions per week and the number of weeks increased. The benefits from the exercise seem to last 2 to 4 hours. (7)

It is obvious that a person who is physically fit will have a better self concept than one who is unfit. This is an important part of a person's total self concept and their self esteem. Since people with better self concepts and higher self esteem are more able to handle stressors, physically fit people should experience fewer negative effects from stressors than those who are unfit. (8) 9)

Exercise activities which have positive outcomes for us are more likely to result in better self concepts. These positive outcomes might be in:

-- success (such as running or swimming faster, or losing weight and developing a more pleasing body shape),

-- increased feeling of physical competence (such as skiing or playing tennis better), or

-- goal attainment (such as lifting a heavier weight, reducing one's resting pulse rate, or shooting a lower golf score).

Effective exercise has also been shown to reduce the illnesses which often accompany stressful events in our lives. (9) Exercisers also report a lower incidence of colon, breast, and prostate cancer. (10)

So it can be seen that exercise is both an effective method of <u>preventing</u> the stronger negative reactions that can result from stressors and a method for <u>reducing</u> those negative reactions when they are present. These are benefits which accrue in addition to the commonly sought outcomes of : weight control, aerobic fitness, strength, muscle definition, and flexibility.

Exercise has been shown to be as effective as other stress management techniques in reducing depression, tension, and anger. (11) Since exercising aerobically (running, swimming, etc.) is inexpensive and takes the same amount of time as other techniques, while giving additional benefits of weight control and cardiovascular fitness, it should be high on everyone's list of necessary daily activities.

Choosing the Coping Technique. Each type of stress may be more effectively handled by the choice of an appropriate coping technique:

--When you are experiencing physical symptoms such as: tense muscles, a rapid heart rate, or a lack of energy, a physical activity may help you to better handle the stress. Running, swimming, cycling, cross country skiing, massage, or yoga may be the better choices for your stress reduction.

--When your stress reactions are mental such as: anxiety, worry, insomnia, and negative thinking about yourself, your better choices for coping may be: meditation, the relaxation response or hypnosis.

--If your stresses are caused by a hectic schedule, having too many things to do and too much responsibility, your better coping mechanisms may be: assertiveness training (to be able to say "no" to some people who want more of your time), time management (to be better able to schedule the important activities), biofeedback, and psychological assistance to change your time pressured type A behavior to a more relaxed mode of living.

Thinking Our Way to Reducing or Eliminating Our Distresses

The ideal method for handling stresses is to not merely "cope" with them but rather to eliminate them--if that is a possibility. Often people just accept a stressor rather than find a way to eliminate the problem. Effective thinking can often aid us in many areas, and eliminating stressors is one very important area. Also, learning to think will help to raise our level of self esteem because it is an important aspect of our evaluation of ourselves. We shouldn't get upset because we made a mistake because making a mistake indicates that you at least tried to do something.

Effective decision making is the sign of a mature, self actualized person. But how do we think? How do we choose wisely? What are the steps to effective thinking and effective problem solving? How can I use the proven thinking techniques to reduce or eliminate problems and stresses in our lives?

The Scientific Method of Problem Solving

The famous American philosopher-psychologist-educator John Dewey can be credited with the approach we will suggest to solving problems. It was his contention that the method of science can be applied to our individual problems; and when applied should make the problems more easily soluble. Here are the steps you might use to solve a problem:

(1) Define the problem
(2) Clarify the problem with facts about it
(3) Look at several possible solutions
(4) Choose the best possible solution
(5) Try it and evaluate its outcome.

Successful use of problem solving can reduce stresses at every age and can even reduce severe depression. (The Menninger Letter, June 1994, p. 6) But as with most techniques which work, it takes thought, time, and commitment. So if you honestly want to make a change in your life, here are the steps.

TAKING CHARGE OF YOUR LIFE

Life never runs completely smoothly. There are always those impediments to happiness-- those stressors in our lives. Often people dwell on the stresses. Their whole lives may be used in making excuses or in retreating from life through drugs, deep depressions, or other unhealthy escapes.

Our lives will all be touched by some negative stressors--disabilities, failures, death, break ups of relationships, and other personal catastrophes. We cannot let these hurdles trip us and stop our race towards a positive, fulfilling, socially useful life. We must learn how to eliminate those stressors which we can and successfully cope with those which we cannot eliminate. As world renowned sport psychologist Tara Scanlan has questioned "Do we want to spend our lives coping or enjoying?"

Perhaps the most famous, and the most succinct, phrasing of our task was enunciated by the German theologian Reinhold Niebuhr in what is called "The Serenity Prayer."

God grant me--
The *serenity* to accept the things I cannot change;
The *courage* to change the things I can; and
The *wisdom* to know the difference.

END NOTES

1. Berger, Bonnie G. "Coping with Stress: The effectiveness of exercise and other techniques. " Paper presented at the Annual Meeting of the American Academy of Kinesiology and Physical Education, March 24, 1993. Published in Quest, vol. 46, 1994

2. Feuerstein, M., Labbe, E.E., , and Kuczmierczyk, A. R. Health Psychology: A psychobiological perspective. New York: Plenum. 1986. p 189

3. Dillbeck, M.C., Orme-Johnson, D.W. Physiological differences between transcendental meditation and rest. American Psychologist. vol. 42. 1987. pp 879-881

4. Bensen, Herbert. The Relaxation Response. William Morrow, New York, 1975.

5. Berger, Bonnie. "Mood Alteration with Exercise: A taxonomy to maximize benefits. Paper presented at the VIII World Congress of Sport Psychology, Lisbon, Portugal, June 23, 1993.

6. Boutcher, S.H. and Landers, D. M. The effects of vigorous exercise on anxiety, heart rate, and alpha activity of runners and non-runners. Psychophysiology, vol. 25, 1988. pp. 696-702

7. Raglin, J.S. and Morgan, W.P. Influences of exercise and quiet rest on state anxiety and blood pressure. Medicine and Science in Sports and Exercise. Vol. 19. 1987. pp 436-463

8. Tucker, L.A. Effect of weight training on body attitudes: who benefits most? Journal of Sports Medicine and Physical Fitness. Vol. 27, 1987, pp 70-78; Young, M. L. Estimation of fitness and physical ability, physical performance, and self-concept among adolescent females. Journal of Sports Medicine and Physical Fitness, Vol. 25. 1985 pp. 144-150.

9. (Brown, J.D. Staying fit and staying well: physical fitness as a moderator of life stress. Journal of Personality and Social Psychology, vol. 60, 1991, pp 555-561.

10. Mackinnon, L. T. Exercise and immunology: current issues in exercise science. [Monograph No. 2] Champaign, IL: Human Kinetics. 1992; Sternfeld, B., Cancer and the protective effect of physical activity: the epidemiological evidence. Medicine and Science in Sports and Exercise. vol. 24. 1991. pp 1195-1209.

11. Berger, B.G., Friedman, E. and Easton, M. "Comparison of jogging, the relaxation response, and group interaction for stress reduction." Journal of Sport and Exercise Psychology, vol. 10, 1988, pp 431-447; Long, B.C. and Haney, C.J. "Coping strategies for working women: Aerobic exercise and relaxation interventions." Behavior Therapy. vol. 19. 1988. pp 75-83; Long and Haney. "Long term follow up of stressed

working women: a comparison of aerobic exercise and progressive relaxation." Journal of Sport and Exercise Psychology. vol. 10. 1988. pp. 461-470.

CHAPTER 18
MEDICAL AND DENTAL AIDS TO HEALTH AND BEAUTY

Our emphasis, up to now, has been making your body under the skin younger and making it possible to live longer. But as you all know, the media attempts to influence us to look young even if our bodies are getting older under our skin. Since plastic surgery and dental techniques can make us look more like the media ideals we're all familiar with, we often opt for such external enhancements. We should be aware of the possibilities and the potential dangers, as well as the financial cost.

Some people seem to go to extremes in terms of what they expect plastic surgery to do and what they want from it. The 80-year-old comedienne, Joan Rivers, is said to have had 700 plastic surgery procedures-- according to her daughter.

Reconstructive surgery, where the body is put back together, is obviously important for most people. A number of people have hand surgery due to injuries in which rings were involved. In fact ring related hand surgeries are a major reconstructive procedure. People who have been burned commonly need some reconstructive surgery. And you probably have heard of the two recent face transplants that have been done successfully. But here we are going to talk about

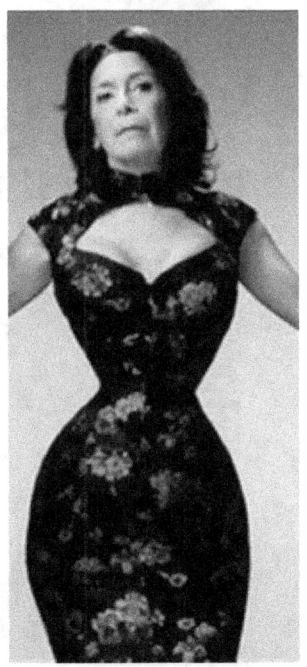

Both men and women are increasingly going under the knife to look a little younger. These procedures usually take away tissue such as in facelift, liposuction or breast reduction. Other procedures add to the existing body, such as breast or other body implants, subdural injections for lip or cheek enhancement or hair implants. There are many of us who are not perfectly content with our bodies. But if we plan plastic surgery to augment our lips, cheeks or muscles we should be certain of what we want and find a competent surgeon to do the procedure.

Take away a few ribs and add some pads to the hips—and you are instantly gorgeous! Take away some wrinkles and add some collagen to the lips and cheeks and you have an unforgetable face!

If you aren't getting big enough—fast enough at the gym, a couple of well placed

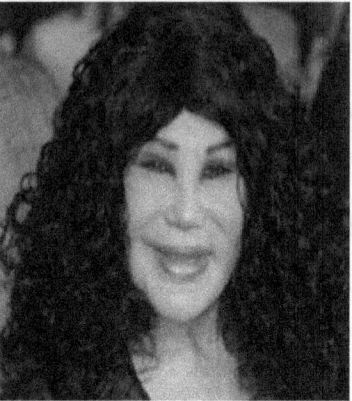

implants will certainly attract the ladies!

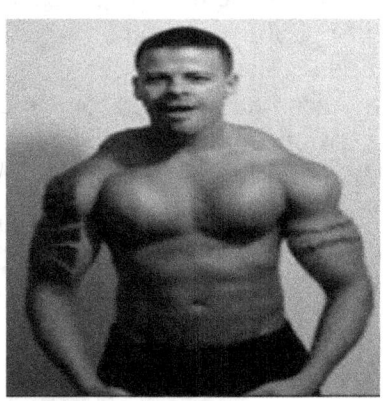

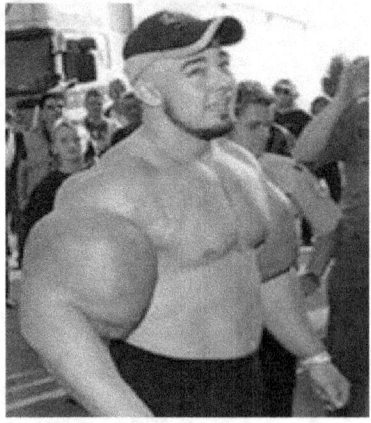

TYPES OF PLASTIC SURGERY PROCEDURES

HEAD-- nose reshaping, cheek augmentation, chin augmentation, ear surgery, eyelid surgery, facelift, facial implants, forehead lift, lip augmentation

BREAST--breast augmentation, breast implants, breast lift, female breast reduction, male breast reduction

SKIN--chemical peel deep, chemical peel light, fat injection, other injectables, laser hair removal, micropigmentation, microdermabrasion

BODY--liposuction, body part enhancements, upper arm reduction, tummy tuck, POST GASTRIC SURGERY (post-bariatric) tummy tuck, skin tightening

The advantages of a selected surgery are obvious (a better looking face or figure, a loss of fat or the reshaping of a less than ideal ear or eyelid) so we will here look at some of the risks of some common procedures.

Breast Augmentation - Breasts are enlarged by placing an implant behind each breast.

Risks: implants can rupture, leak, and deflate; infection; hardening of scar tissue around implant, causing breast firmness, pain, distorted shape, or implant movement; bleeding; pain; nipples may get more or less sensitive; numbness near incision blood collection around implant/incision; calcium deposits around implant; harder to find breast lumps (possible cancer indicators)

Breast Lift - Extra skin is removed from the breast to raise and reshape breast.

Risks: scarring; skin loss; infection loss of feeling in nipples or breast; nipples put in the wrong place; breasts not symmetrical

Breast Reduction - Fat, tissue, and skin is removed from breast.

Risks: if nipples and areola are detached, may lose sensation and decreased ability to breastfeed; bleeding; infection; scarring; harder to find breast lumps; poor shape, size, or position of nipples or breasts

Eyelid Surgery: Extra fat, skin, and muscle in the upper and/or lower eyelid is removed to correct "droopy" eyelids.

Risks: blurred or double vision; infection; bleeding under the skin; swelling; dry eyes, whiteheads; can't close eye completely; pulling of lower lids; blindness

Facelift - Extra fat is removed, muscles are tightened, and skin is rewrapped around the face and neck to improve sagging facial skin, jowls, and loose neck skin.

Risks: infection; bleeding under skin; scarring; irregular earlobes; nerve damage causing numbness or inability to move your face; skin damage; loss of some hair

Facial Implant - infection feeling of tightness or scarring around implant shifting of implant

Risks: infection; feeling of tightness or scarring around implant; shifting of implant

Forehead Lift: Extra skin and muscles that cause wrinkles are removed, eyebrows are lifted, and forehead skin is tightened.

Risks: eye dryness or irritation; infection; scarring; bleeding under skin ; impaired eyelid function; loss of feeling in eyelid skin; injury to facial nerve causing loss of motion or muscle weakness

Lip Augmentation: Material is injected or implanted into the lips to create fuller lips and reduce wrinkles around the mouth.

Risks: infection; bleeding; lip asymmetry; lumping; scarring

Liposuction: Excess fat from a targeted area is removed with a vacuum to shape the body.

Risks: baggy skin; skin may change color and fall off; fluid retention; shock; infection; fat clots in the lungs; pain; damage to organs if punctured; numbness at the surgery site; heart problems; kidney problems; disability; death

Nose Surgery: Nose is reshaped by resculpting the bone and cartilage in the nose.

Risks: infection; bursting blood vessels; red spots; bleeding under the skin; scarring

Tummy Tuck: Extra fat and skin in the abdomen is removed, and muscles are tightened to flatten tummy.

Risks: infection; blood clots: bleeding; scarring; fluid accumulation under the skin

EXTENT OF PLASTIC PROCEDURES

There were over 9 million surgical and nonsurgical cosmetic procedures in the US last year. 18% of these are surgical and accounted for 63% of the total expenditures. Since 1997 there has been about a 200% increase in cosmetic procedures. People in the 35 to 60 age range have most of the procedures--43%. In the 19 to 34 age group, they had 20% of the procedures and the over-60 group had 36%.

American men had more than 750,000 cosmetic procedures in 2010, according to ASAPS statistics. While that number represents just 8 percent of the total, the number of annual cosmetic procedures for men has increased more than 88 percent since 1997. Nearly 75 percent of those procedures were for men between the ages of 35 and 64.

The top five surgical procedures for men in 2011 were: liposuction (42,000), nose changes (rhinoplasty) (25,000), eyelid surgery (23,000), breast reduction to treat enlarged male breasts (17,000), and facelifts (10,000). Cosmetic ear surgery (10,000) was sixth. Hair transplantation was also high on the list. The tummy tuck is also a fast-rising procedure that will likely crack the top five soon.

For women it was: breast augmentation 320,000, liposuction 283,000, tummy tuck 43,000, eyelid surgery 125,000, and breast lifts 127,000.

The top nonsurgical procedures were Botox and other wrinkle removing techniques. with nearly 4 million procedures. Laser hair removal with nearly 1,000,000 procedures micro dermal abrasion with a half million.

Women had 91% of the total procedures. The top surgical procedures for women were: breast augmentation, liposuction, breast lifts, and eyelid surgery. For men they were: liposuction, nose procedures, eyelid surgery, breast reduction and facelifts.

MINIMALLY INVASIVE PROCEDURES

Minimally invasive procedures include: injections for wrinkle removal, hair removal and skin peels. Some soft tissue fillers, such as lip enhancements, are also included. Botox (botulinum Toxin Type A) was used 4,030,318 times last year. Hyaluronic Acid has primary uses in joint pain reduction and eye surgeries but it is now also used in wrinkle reduction. Restylane is a trade name in cosmetic circles. It was used 1,662,480 times last year. Laser hair removal was done nearly a million and a half times. Skin peeling was done about 800,000 times and IPL (Intense Pulsed Light) treatments over 700,000 times. There are many contraindications and some horror stories associated with IPL treatments.

WRINKLE REDUCTION

Wrinkle reduction is generally handled by a muscle relaxant that slows or eliminates the contractions of some muscles just below the skin that cause some wrinkles. Botox is such a chemical. There are also fillers that replace the fat that has been lost as we age. Some of these are permanent and some wear off in a few months. And of course there is a surgical procedure of facelift.

BOTOX®(onabotulinumtoxinA) is the result of more than 100 years of study into botulinum toxin type A

BOTOX is used in a number of conditions in which a neurotoxin can be valuable, including turning some migraine sufferers and some of the problems attending the multiple sclerosis. It works by blocking some purpose impulses that elicit muscle contractions.

RISKS

We know why you want a procedure, but with every surgery, injection or gel there are occasionally unforeseen problems. So here are some possible risks to these procedures.

Botox Injection: Botox is injected into a facial muscle to paralyze it, so lines don't form when a person frowns or squints.

Risks: face pain; muscle weakness; flu-like symptoms; headaches; loss of facial expression; droopy eyelids; asymmetric smile; drooling

Collagen/fat Injection: Collagen from a cow or fat from your thigh or abdomen is injected into facial wrinkles, pits, or scars.

Risks: it may trigger an autoimmune disease; the contours may not come out as you desired: contour problems; hives or rash, swelling; flu-like symptoms

Dermabrasion: A small, spinning wheel or brush with a roughened surface removes the upper layers of facial skin. A new layer of skin appears during healing, giving the face a smoother appearance. Used to treat facial scars, heavy wrinkles, and problems like rosacea.

Risks: abnormal color changes; infection; whiteheads; fever blisters or cold sores; allergic reactions; thickened skin

Hyaluronic acid injection: This gel is injected into your face to smooth lines, wrinkles, and scars on the skin.

Risks: swelling; redness or infection; lumps; tissue hardening; lumps under the skin

Laser hair removal: Laser light is passed over the skin to remove hair.

Risks: change in skin color, scarring, regrowth of hair

Laser skin resurfacing: Laser light is used to remove wrinkles, lines, age spots, scars, , tattoos, moles and warts from the surface of the skin.

Risks: scarring; burning; change in skin color, herpes flare up

Unsightly vein treatments (sclerotherapy) A solution is injected into spider and varicose leg veins (small purple and red blood vessels) to remove the veins.

Risks: may not be permanent; blood clotting; skin color changes; scarring

Chemical Peel: A solution is put onto the face (or parts of the face) that causes the skin to blister and peel off. It is replaced with new skin.

Risks: scarring; infection; cold sores; heart problems, allergic reaction

Tooth Whiteners (peroxide agents): Depending on the product, either you or the dentist applies peroxide using strips; a mouth guard with gel; or a tray inside your mouth around your teeth

Risks: If not customized for you by a dentist or dental hygienist, there may be unknown ingredients and unknown results. (1)

OTHER SURGICAL PROCEDURES

Stomach stapling or gastric by-pass may be ways of reducing the accumulation of calories that have settled as fat. Such surgeries may have very positive results—but the risks are significant. For example there is a 16% chance of nerve damage and pain, according to a Mayo Clinic study. These were at least partially related to malnutrition. Such weight loss surgeries are not recommended unless the BMI is in the 35 to 40% range.

DENTAL PROCEDURES

Dental procedures most commonly utilized by adults are: tooth whitening, tooth capping and straightening teeth. The whitening is simply done with the aid of a dentist along with commercially available whitening toothpastes or gels. Capping and straightening teeth must be done by a dentist. There are some modern ways of straightening teeth without our both faster and less visible than the traditional metal braces.

END NOTES

1. The National Women's Health Information Center (www4woman.gov)

For more information on various surgical procedures check this link and find the procedure that you have question about.

http://www.surgery.org/consumers/procedures/body/

EPILOGUE

The habits we have that will make us live long usually also make us look younger. Tighter muscles, better posture, slimmer bodies and a healthier diet not only extend our lives but also make us feel better about ourselves. As our lifespans extend we may opt for the medical advances that can help our outsides match our insides. The key to real happiness, however, is a sound mind in a sound body. So as we age we want to keep our minds active and productive-- just as we do for our bodies.

www.ingramcontent.com/pod-product-compliance
Lightning Source LLC
Chambersburg PA
CBHW080411290526
45791CB00008BA/2234